"Caroline Leaf marvelously addresses the single most important issue of our lives—that we can learn to control our brains, take charge of our minds, and improve how we feel, think, and live. We do not need psychiatric medications: we need knowledge, reason, and love to move beyond our suffering to lead fulfilling lives."

Peter R. Breggin, MD, psychiatrist
and author of *Guilt, Shame and Anxiety*

"I first encountered Dr. Caroline Leaf's work by observing how her *Switch On Your Brain* book, with its 5-Step Learning Process, took my husband, Peter, from despair to hope in his neuroscience graduate program. I have also since recognized the applicability of her work for children's educational success and focus. Even our own son appreciates its utility with school work. I believe the content of this book is revolutionary. In my eighteen years of practice as an obstetrician and gynecologist, predominantly providing care for patients in inner-city communities, I come across many women who may be considered without hope. Many seem to be stuck in a cycle of poverty, with its untoward effects on family, often seeing themselves as victims. I believe once they get a hold of this book, read it, and apply it, they will realize there is power in their minds to change not just their own lives but the lives of their children and their communities. As a famous Ghanaian educator Dr. James Kwegir-Aggrey once said, 'If you educate a man you educate an individual, but if you educate a woman you educate a nation.'"

Mercy Amua-Quarshie, MD, MPH, diplomate
of the American Board of Obstetrics and Gynecology

"Dr. Leaf helps us develop healthy thoughts, and her scientifically researched and clinically applied work illuminates the way we live, love, and learn. The techniques and exercises in this book will benefit you in school, work, and your relationships!"

David I. Levy, MD, clinical professor of neurosurgery
and author of *Gray Matter*

D0250516

"In nearly thirty years as a neurologist, I have witnessed a global shift in the 'way' we are thinking, along with an epidemic decrease in our overall mental health and an epidemic increase in neurophysiologically disruptive disorders. Consequently, I believe this new text by Dr. Leaf should be a required read-and-study for all of us who want to think, learn, and succeed—this is a message of practical hope that is a scientifically based program of action."

Robert P. Turner, MD, MSCR, QEEGD, BCN, associate professor of clinical pediatrics and neurology, University of South Carolina School of Medicine and Palmetto Health Richland Children's Hospital; associate researcher, MIND Research Institute, Irvine, California

"Wow! Another amazing book written by Dr. Leaf! In simple terms, she effectively describes how complex neurophysiological processes can either help or impair your success in life. It is so exciting to see Dr. Leaf nailing down several misconceptions and myths in the medical world. Paraphrasing a truth I learned from her, we are not a product of our own biology. We have brilliant minds that help us transform the barriers we face into stepping stones, leading us to a place where we can reach our full potential—not through excessive or unhealthy work schedules but by being mindful in everything we do, from the thoughts we think to the foods we eat to the ways we work and rest. As an endocrinologist, I see how 'toxic' thinking affects my patients on a daily basis. Oftentimes, this thinking is a huge barrier stopping them from being able to maintain their well-being, restore their health, or achieve their goals. My hope is that everyone, especially patients with endocrine dysfunctions, will read this amazing collection of life-giving, truthful information! Understanding the wisdom Dr. Leaf is sharing can make a huge difference in changing your life for the better."

Irinel Stanciu, MD, fellow of the American College of Endocrinology

"No matter your situation in life, you have the power to make positive changes. Dr. Leaf has done a masterful job of describing how different mindsets, through quantum effects, change our brains. Through simple steps outlined in this book, you can change your brain and experience a successful life. So don't stay stuck in defeat—apply the steps in this book and experience the triumphant life!"

Timothy R. Jennings, MD, DFAPA, former president
of the Tennessee and Southern Psychiatric Association
and author of *The Aging Brain*

"The brilliant Dr. Caroline Leaf travels 'beyond mindfulness' in this landmark work, giving the tools to developing meaningful cognitive transformation in order to succeed! She rightly dismisses neuro-myths that are taken for truth in our current society, similar to what is encountered in the physician-patient interaction after superficial web search–level knowledge has to be put in context. We also see a rise in fatalities due to OUD (opioid use disorders) and SUD (substance use disorders) at epidemic proportions in our nation. These disorders stem in part from past physical and emotional trauma that we are all subject to. The salient points brought to light by Dr. Leaf give us insight into how these habits are formed in the disordered mind. She also gives us hope by bringing to light God's methodology to address the very origin of the outward manifestation of these "mind" problems. Another triumphant work, Dr. Leaf!"

Avery M. Jackson, neurosurgeon, CEO, and founder
of the Michigan Neurosurgical Institute PC

"As Dr. Caroline Leaf's former professor for her Masters and PhD degrees, research mentor, and longtime friend, I am delighted and excited to see how the research on the mind-brain connection and cognitive neuroscience she began with her degrees as a communication pathologist has developed into an extraordinary book that will help people think, learn, and succeed in every area of their lives. This well-researched book not only shows individuals how much power they have in their minds but how to use this power wisely. Not only has Caroline applied these scientifically researched concepts successfully in her clinical practice, educational, and corporate spheres but she has also applied this approach in her own personal life and with her family—so her latest book needs no more validation than her own success story!"

Dr. Brenda Louw, professor and chair, Speech-Language
Pathology and Audiology, East Tennessee State University

"Dr. Caroline Leaf is an incredible gift to us all! In her new book, *Think, Learn, Succeed*, she unlocks and reveals the wisdom and science behind how we process information to understand how we individually think! This is the golden ticket! With her research, revealed in this book, we can now unleash our full potential and get beyond the fog that comes with not thinking clearly or successfully. This is the answer for the student who struggles with learning and retaining information and the executive who deals with anxiety before that big board presentation. . . . I firmly believe, as a medical doctor, that *Think, Learn, Succeed* can make the difference in our personal health—cognitive and physical. This book has the potential to make a real difference in dementia and cognitive decline. The mind changes the brain, and I know this book will do just that for you. This book is a must-have, must-read, must-do! I wish I had this book when I was going though medical school, and I will definitely recommend it to my patients and anyone who is a student! In fact, I use all of Dr. Leaf's books in my practice and recommend them to my patients because they work."

Jason Littleton, MD, chairman of Family Medicine
at Orlando Regional Medical Center and
founder and CEO of Littleton Concierge Medicine

"Dr. Leaf has an amazing mind and a special gift of communication. As a counselor and someone who helps lead counselors internationally, I cannot recommend *Think, Learn, Succeed* enough! It is a powerful resource that shows people how much they are able to help themselves by giving individuals both the knowledge and the resources to change the way they think, thereby changing the way they live their lives."

Dr. Tim Clinton, president of the American Association
of Christian Counselors

"Dr. Leaf's work has had a tremendous impact on my life. In 2015, I was severely depressed and had many panic attacks. I exhausted myself going from one psychiatrist to another, to no avail. Through Dr. Leaf's research, I found the resources that completely healed me and changed my life and the lives of others. What is most striking about *Think, Learn, Succeed* is how Dr. Leaf is so driven with a passion to encourage each of us recognize how powerful we really are and how much can be conquered if only we get our minds right—diseases, hardships, and crises can be overcome with the power of the mind. In *Think, Learn, Succeed*, she gives us a practical guide to help us grow into the mindsets that will bring us abundance in life. In this book, you will find Dr. Leaf bringing a bold proposition to the table: a new paradigm that can bring about a true revolution in wellbeing and healthcare. I am confident that we're about to enter a new phase of healthcare that will be led by her Dr. Leaf's research and resources. We've been asking ourselves what could happen if we were to build a system that is not focused on the disease; I strongly believe Dr. Leaf already knows the answer, and we as an organization are fiercely joining forces with her to accelerate her vision."

Igor P. Morais, doctor of dental surgery, University of Brasília,
Brazil, and researcher in oral surgery and public healthcare

"Dr. Leaf provides a pedagogical approach to living a fulfilling life. As you read through the pages of her book, you become her student, discovering how your mindset may be keeping you stagnant in life and learning her methods, proven over decades of scientific research and application, to change it. She reveals how negative thoughts subtly hijack our minds through various life experiences, becoming the blueprint by which we build our lives. This book exposes the destructive nature of unhealthy thoughts and teaches you how to harness the power of your own mind, unlocking your ability to learn information you may have found intimidating or impossible. It transcends all walks of life, including college students looking to perform better on exams, professionals wanting to excel in their careers, stay-at-home parents desiring to function with more clarity, and retirees trying to stave off or mitigate the effects of Alzheimer's. As with embarking on any meaningful journey, her methods do not offer a quick solution but they do offer a guaranteed and long-lasting one if you put in the work. I charge you with the assignment of reading this book if you are looking to free your mind of chaotic and unproductive thinking, increase your IQ, and take command of your life."

Lillian Lockett Robertson, MD, OB/GYN, FACOG

"*Think, Learn, Succeed* addresses many issues we struggle with in today's school environment. If I can sum this book up into one overarching theme, I would say this book helps to teach 'personal responsibility.' Dr. Leaf brings a unique approach to learning. From the chapters on mindset, the gift profile, and the 5-step learning process, she makes it is so easy to understand and teaches it in a very concrete way. Every chapter in this book is extremely necessary for today's learners, especially in the public school environment, where fear and loneliness may try to take control of students' thought life. Not only does this book help teach students to think and learn but it also pulls in the very important aspects of a healthy lifestyle, especially in building positive mindsets. This is the start to developing students' goal-setting and dream-building, which is an important aspect in our schools. Many students lack a sense of purpose and come from toxic environments. They do not understand how their learning in school and in life is impacted by their own thinking, mood, and emotions. This book makes it clear how to create changes for every aspect of our mind, body, and emotions and addresses the need to be explicitly taught. I also love the activation tips that are placed at the end of each chapter, which provide easy and reasonable ways to activate learning. As educators, we know that if we do not have an end-product to learning, the learning remains in short-term memory and will not be sustained."

Angela McDonald, MA, superintendent and
CEO of Advantage Academy

THINK,
LEARN,
SUCCEED

THINK, LEARN, SUCCEED

Understanding and Using Your Mind to
Thrive at School, the Workplace, and Life

DR. CAROLINE LEAF

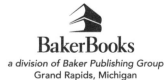

BakerBooks
a division of Baker Publishing Group
Grand Rapids, Michigan

Published by Baker Books
a division of Baker Publishing Group
PO Box 6287, Grand Rapids, MI 49516-6287
www.bakerbooks.com

Paperback edition published 2019
ISBN 978-0-8010-9468-2

Printed in the United States of America

The Library of Congress has cataloged the original edition as follows:
Names: Leaf, Caroline, 1963– author.
Title: Think, learn, succeed : understanding and using your mind to thrive at school, the workplace, and life / Dr. Caroline Leaf.
Description: Grand Rapids : Baker Publishing Group, 2018.
Identifiers: LCCN 2018007039 | ISBN 9780801093272 (cloth)
Subjects: LCSH: Thought and thinking. | Psychology.
Classification: LCC BF441 .L394 2018 | DDC 158.1—dc23
LC record available at https://lccn.loc.gov/2018007039

9780801093616 (ITPE)

The Switch On Your Brain 5-Step Learning Process and The Metacog are registered trademarks of Dr. Caroline Leaf.

This publication is intended to provide helpful and informative material on the subjects addressed. Readers should consult their personal health professionals before adopting any of the suggestions in this book or drawing inferences from it. The author and publisher expressly disclaim responsibility for any adverse effects arising from the use or application of the information contained in this book.

19 20 21 22 23 24 25   7 6 5 4 3 2 1

This book is dedicated to *everyone*, because everyone needs to think, learn, and succeed in school, work, and life!

Let's stop *striving* and let's start *thriving*—together!

Out of the night that covers me,
    Black as the pit from pole to pole,
I thank whatever gods may be
    For my unconquerable soul.

In the fell clutch of circumstance
    I have not winced nor cried aloud.
Under the bludgeonings of chance
    My head is bloody, but unbowed.

Beyond this place of wrath and tears
    Looms but the Horror of the shade,
And yet the menace of the years
    Finds and shall find me unafraid.

It matters not how strait the gate,
    How charged with punishments the scroll,
I am the master of my fate,
    I am the captain of my soul.

— William Ernest Henley, "Invictus"

Contents

Foreword

Just over ten years ago I was in a very tight spot. I had to take an all-day written exam in the neuroscience graduate program I was in. No one I knew had passed that exam, and those who had failed were basically kicked off the program. It seemed clear to me there was a conspiracy to force me off the program, due to a series of previous events.

Studying the vast amount of information was not going well for me—I was very frustrated and losing hope. I could not sleep well. I was in this state of mind when, one night about 2:00 a.m., I was flipping through TV channels and came across Dr. Leaf being interviewed on a talk show. What caught my attention was the eloquence with which she was able to explain how the brain works in practical terms. I was a neuroscience student and already a medical doctor, and what she said made sense to me. When I found out from her website she had developed a process that had helped many thousands of students around the world excel in their studies, hope started to fill my heart. I dared to ask—Could I possibly pass the impassable? As I began to use the Switch On Your Brain 5-Step Learning Process and its tool, the Metacog, from what I could glean from her website and her book (which I later ordered from South Africa), I knew the answer to my question was a resounding yes!

After passing the exam by using her methods, and leaving that program with a master's in neuroscience, I have collaborated with Dr. Leaf ever since.

Dr. Leaf has written some great books over the years; however, I must confess, this is my favorite for many reasons. First, it was the material in this book that saved my academic career. Second, I have taught students from high school to graduate school using the principles in this book and have seen their academic and emotional lives change. Third, the principles in this book have helped my own family. And finally, this is my favorite Caroline Leaf book because of highly emotional reasons that go way back to 1976, when I was about twelve years old. That was the year of the Soweto school riots in South Africa, an event that shocked the world. I looked with horror at pictures of children carrying their dead and injured friends from the line of fire. Years later Dr. Caroline Leaf worked for twenty-plus years in the townships, including Soweto, and dramatically changed hundreds of schools and hundreds of thousands of students through the principles, processes, and techniques explained in this book.

In this book, Dr. Leaf lays out a roadmap to success in our schools and colleges, the workplace, and our personal lives. I suggest you read the book in the order she has laid out, because each principle and process builds on the previous one. There is no quick fix or shortcut. I encourage you, dear reader, to stay the course—I believe the journey will be well worth it, not just for you but for subsequent generations as well.

There are profound changes taking place in classrooms, workplaces, and businesses around the world. Information is increasing at an exponential rate; however, the management of information has not kept pace. Information overload is not just negatively affecting our effectiveness but our mental health as well. I believe this book offers a timely solution to the problem.

Peter Amua-Quarshie, MD, MPH, MS,
assistant professor of basic medical sciences

Prologue

Everyone seems to be talking about mindfulness and taking the time to invest in yourself. But how do you really make your mind work for you? How do you use your mind to shape your life? How do you "invest" in yourself, creating a lifestyle that promotes both brain and body health? How do you go beyond awareness of, calming down, and acknowledging feelings, thoughts, and bodily sensations in the present moment to making sustainable, long-lasting changes? You are the "captain of your soul," after all!

It is easy to say you want to take care of yourself, but how do you take care of the mind, which takes care of everything else? The answer is not some pill, diet fad, magic number, Instagram account with over a million followers, or some quick-fix memory program. We all have significant resources at our fingertips. Our minds are incredibly powerful—we can use our thoughts to improve our overall intellect, cognitive performance, and mental and physical well-being. Harnessing these natural resources will give you power over your present, depth and context to your past, and anticipation for the future.

How you *understand and use* your mind is predictive of how successful you will be. We all think, feel, and choose in unique ways;

we all define our own meaningful success. This book is all about helping you get to that place where you succeed in all these key areas and make that switch to a life that is well-lived and filled with *meaningful* success. This book is about mental self-care. It takes you beyond mindfulness into a lifestyle of cognitive transformation that is both sustainable and organic—suited to your *Perfect You*.[1]

Mental self-care is integrally interwoven into a life of meaning, which naturally evolves into success in school, work, and every other area of your life. It is the key to finding your vocation: what gets you out of bed in the morning, and every morning to come. You can only be you, and who you are is brilliant, exciting, and inspiring.

Indeed, many years of research and many thousands of people later, I am still taken aback by the power of our minds to

- learn effectively
- change circumstances
- increase creativity
- improve memory and its functionality
- increase emotional control, allowing emotions and stress to work for you and not against you
- experience intellectual satisfaction

Whether you are at school and just want to learn how to learn, whether you are in corporate life and need to improve your memory and performance, whether you are a stay-at-home or working parent juggling professional and personal responsibilities, whether you feel your mind and memory are not functioning as they should—you need this book because you are a thinking, learning being. You are always thinking and learning, every moment of every day. The questions we need to ask, then, are: *What* should I think and learn? *How* should I think and learn?

Are you thinking and learning to *succeed*?

In this book, I will provide you with three practical, scientific mental self-care tools to help you develop successful thinking and learning habits and achieve sustainable, long-lasting change in your life. I have researched, developed, and presented these three tools over thirty years to hundreds of thousands of people around the world and have been amazed at the results:

- *The Mindset Guide*—a practical guide that will give you insight into the power of how mindsets can change your brain and develop cognitive resilience, which is essential to success.
- *The Gift Profile*—a tool to find your customized thinking—the unique way you process information to understand how you think. Understanding how you think will activate the power of mindsets, turning them from being "nice to know about" into real, driving forces of change in your life. Stop talking and start doing.
- *The Switch On Your Brain 5-Step Learning Process*—a technique to build memory and learn successfully, based on how the mind processes information through the brain. The brain is designed to grow constantly, and the power of mindsets can really only energize sustainable, successful change when we think in our customized ways and build useful memory.

Mindsets contain power; customized thinking activates this power; the five-step process builds this power into long-term sustainable change. So, these powerful tools can help you improve your memory, learning, cognitive and intellectual performance, work performance, physical performance, relationships, and emotional health.

You will shift your life from survival mode to success mode!

Acknowledgments

When I wrote the first draft of this book and gave it to my team, waxing on excitedly about how "Microtubules and tubulin as neurobiological quantum computers explain how, in my Geodesic Information Processing Model (the theory and research I developed thirty years ago), memory is essentially seen as part of the cognitive process, where the new descriptive systems are reconceptualized or redesigned," they politely looked at each other and then me, and said, "No one except you and your academic colleagues are going to read that." And this was six weeks before the manuscript due date.

What happened next was an amazing experience and ended up producing my best work—this book, the seventeenth book I have written.

Dominique, one of my team (and my second daughter, a Pepperdine graduate with experience working in Hollywood), sat me down and said very directly, "Mom, what are you trying to say? I have grown up with your scientific thinking and learning methods and they work; they are revolutionary. You are a mind specialist, but what you have just explained is too complex." And so began a day-long discussion with many notes being written as Dominique, with insightful brilliance, drew the best out of me, and six weeks later my manuscript was transformed into something even my four children (and greatest and most honest critics) loved!

And then my eldest daughter, Jessica, a master's student in the history of theology, stepped in to perform her exceptional and powerful editing magic, and the end result—well, even I want to read it! Thank you, my girls, for your beyond-phenomenal support and genius.

By this stage, this book had become a family affair because my four children were brought up living and using the principles and techniques you will read about in this book. My son, Jeffrey, who is an English major at UCLA, weighed in with some excellent ideas and helped with the title; my youngest daughter, Alexy, who is studying human biology and society at UCLA, offered pearls of wisdom about what her friends and classmates would need from a book like this, and my exceptional and outstanding husband, Mac, my cheerleader and greatest fan, read every word with the marvelous acumen he brings from all his years of being in the corporate environment.

I tell you all of this for the following reason: this book is a family affair, and you are part of the family now because you are reading this book. We are a community wired for love to think, learn, and succeed in school, work, and life—and we help each other achieve this.

As I weave science and life concepts together in this book, I draw on my research and extensive clinical, educational, and corporate experience—and I therefore also want to acknowledge my professors and mentors, especially Prof. Brenda Louw, who honed my scientific and research skills and has been a friend for thirty years. I also acknowledge each and every patient, client, and person I have ever worked with, and everyone who has read my materials, seen me at conferences, or watched and listened to me on TV, YouTube, and my podcasts. Your feedback is invaluable, because you are part of this family as well, and you have helped me understand and work to refine the concepts and techniques I teach in this book.

I also acknowledge the Baker team, who are so integral to the success of disseminating my books to the world. Chad, Mark, Karen, Patti, Lindsey, Erin, Colette, Dave, and the rest of the team: I acknowledge your expertise, professionalism, and guidance over all these years of working together, and I am excited about the future!

Introduction

Are You Succeeding or Just Surviving?

Today, most people can access vast amounts of information, yet few people know how to process this information and use it to be successful at school, work, and life. There is an ever-increasing gap between the "what" (information) and the "how" (the management of information). Our ability to process and understand information has been both encouraged and challenged by the technological revolution. We now have the world at our fingertips, yet, paradoxically, more and more of us live solitary, futile lives. As a result, problems in schools, universities, corporations, institutions, and personal lives abound as we lose sight of the power of mindsets, how to think, and how to learn. This is a global "mental health" issue!

Learning difficulties, inept socialization, mental ill-health, and loneliness, which is purported to be nearing epidemic proportions globally and causing more deaths annually than obesity,[1] compel us to reevaluate our thinking skills and rediscover the notion of community wisdom and the purpose of learning, as opposed to merely gaining pieces of random information to get an A that will make our parents proud or give us a hollow sense of self-worth.

27

A 140-character Twitter post, for instance, can consume inordinate amounts of time, yet no deep thinking ensues: no true satisfaction of mind is attained. Do we understand the damage this is doing? Can we counter it?

When we gather information like puzzle pieces without putting the puzzle together, intellectual growth is stifled. This is a crisis of quantity over quality, and the consequences are frighteningly evident in society. The developed world currently faces a *purported* ADHD epidemic,[2] for instance, where thousands of people, young and old, struggle to concentrate, to learn, to remember, and to think deeply. Thousands of individuals of all ages are being incorrectly labeled as biologically wanting and are medicated with brain damaging substances.[3] Rather than asking what is wrong with our society and the kind of thinking it promotes, we place the blame squarely on an individual's shoulders—or more to the point, their brain—divorcing him or her from the context of daily life.

Indeed, today we are quick to label issues as a disease or disorder rather than applying wisdom and examining what is actually happening in our societies, from the big picture to the detail.[4] In such an environment, it is easy to fear the perils of automation and artificial intelligence (AI), which are no longer merely the concern of Silicon Valley trend watchers—even scholars at Oxford University are making dire predictions.[5] Yet according to a growing body of research, we are asking the wrong questions. The problem is not so much about automation taking over our jobs (and our minds) but rather automation (including seeing humans as biological automatons, or *dehumanization*) changing how we think—and obviously, not always for the better.[6]

How is the technological revolution affecting our ability to think, learn, socialize, and manage the normal day-to-day life of being human? Indeed, what actually constitutes "work" in this day and age? Is the way we're working, working? What are we learning? What is the point of education? Is our thinking changing?

For example, using digital platforms such as tablets and laptops for reading may make us more inclined to focus on concrete details rather than interpreting information more abstractly.[7] This affects reading comprehension and problem-solving.

According to the World Economic Forum, in a 2013 survey of twelve thousand professionals by the *Harvard Business Review*, around 50 percent said they felt their job had no "meaning and significance."[8] What makes knowledge significant? What makes work a vocation? Why do we generally ask people *what* they do but not *why* they do it? How do we get from A, knowledge, to B, significance? Although such questions may seem daunting, compelling us to find the needle of wisdom in a haystack of information, we ask these questions because we are human.

The point of thinking, learning, education, technology, medicine, and philosophy should be to build a better world, with connectedness and humanness as its core fundamental purpose. As journalist Rutger Bregman so eloquently said in his TED talk, "I believe in a future where the point of education is not to prepare you for another useless job but for a life well lived."[9] This is *mental self-care*—a life well-lived, a life of success. The quest for the "good life" is a quest humans have undertaken for millennia. Can you honestly say you have no desire to find out what the "good life" means for you?

We need to recognize that neither society nor our brains are the only factors in determining what we do with our lives. We need to also recognize that our *own* thoughts can hinder our ability to think, learn, and succeed beyond the limits of any society. Have you ever scrolled through Instagram, paralyzed by the feeling that your life somehow doesn't "measure up"? Have you ever felt swamped at work, a crazy "devil wears Prada" boss shouting down at you in an endless, meaningless cycle, because you felt that was the kind of job a responsible adult had to have, that this was what you were supposed to do? Have you ever felt lost preparing for an exam you knew you were going to fail? Sometimes we can be our own worst enemy! Do you just feel like every day you are being hit by something else you need to deal with?

You may feel you don't have any power over your life or circumstances, but you do! Your ability to think, feel, and choose is innately powerful and resilient—you have a mind that is more potent than all the smartphones on the planet combined! You *can* move from survival to success—and it all begins in your mind. In recognizing both the impact of your sociocultural context and your own thoughts, you can redefine your past, reimagine your present, and realize your future.

Neurocentricity and Neuromyths: Incorrect Solutions

We need to get out of the laboratory and off social media and realize we live in dynamic, complex, evolving societies—societies that need each one of us and what we each bring to the table. It is time to introduce the notion of *lifestyle* into the world of education, work, and life. We need to acknowledge the unique nature of thinking and learning within and between specific contexts and cultures—among both communities and individuals.

In recent years, in an attempt to address these modern challenges to thinking and learning, neuroscience has become very popular. It is almost as though adding the prefix "neuro," as in neuroeducation, neuroleadership, neurospirituality, and so on, gives the method, course, program, or book more clout, thereby increasing its credibility. Consequently, several "neuromyths" have arisen out of this neurocentric approach, stifling instead of enhancing human creativity and imagination. A myth satisfies the desire for quick, unequivocal, and simple explanations, and has the potential for the genesis of false ideas and faulty interpretations, which are used and abused by mass media, whose influence in forming and perpetuating opinions is critical.

Reducing the complex nature of humanity to seemingly simplistic neurobiological explanations, in the attempt to address the needs of society at large, is such an example and is not a solution. This type of thinking leads to misperceptions, and thus mismanagement, of learning and education.[10] Furthermore, we ought to be concerned with how we think on an individual, national, and international level, because slick marketing and politicians are able to manipulate an ignorant populace through myths, thereby manipulating the backbone of a democratic system of government.

But what are "neuromyths" specifically? They are common and damaging misconceptions about the nature of brain research, which relate to and shape our understanding of learning, education, work, science, and life. Researchers have surveyed educators, the general public, and people who have completed neuroscience courses to assess their belief in neuromyths.[11] Their research revealed that neuromyth beliefs are remarkably prevalent among the general public, educators, and even neuroscientists (training in neuroscience does not necessarily translate to psychology or education!), hence the potential for interpretive errors to creep in, doing more harm than good.[12] For example, many neuromyths mistakenly imply that a single factor is responsible for a given outcome when learning. However, what these approaches reflect is a gross underestimation of the complexity of human behavior, especially the cognitive and metacognitive skills of attention, reasoning, memory, and learning—which drive the processes of life.[13]

Interestingly, the most commonly endorsed myth from this survey was that individuals learn better when they receive information in their preferred learning style. In chapters 17 and 18, I explain in depth why and how this is wrong, providing a more scientific and logical explanation for how we as individuals uniquely think in our own customized ways. I have been teaching and researching on this for thirty years.

Science, of course, advances through trial and error. A theory is constructed; new phenomena confirm, modify, or refute this theory. Unfortunately, the "messy" advance of science is the only one possible, and invalidated hypotheses always have the potential to turn into myths. Although these beliefs are subsequently demolished by the social process of science, they still have the potential to be widely believed and relayed, and even used by various corporate entities and institutions to promote a specific worldview or agenda.

I have been coming up against these neuromyths all my working and research life. Two neuromyths, in particular, that I have spent three decades teaching against are the left-right brain theory and the learning styles theory, hence my joy in Kelly Macdonald and Lauren McGrath's neuromyth research.[14] Further common myths they identified were the Mozart effect, dyslexia, using ten percent of the brain, and how sugar affects attention. They also found that these "classic" neuromyths tend to cluster together, so if you believe one myth, you are more likely to believe others. I found this to be the case, as well, in my research with educators and mental health professionals. It was a challenge to change their neuromyth mindsets.[15]

Neuromyths about memory abound as well. Memory is not only the heart of learning but is also indispensable in every area of life. It has become the privileged subject of fantasies and false ideas. "Improve Your Memory!" "Increase Your Memory Capacity!" "How to Get an Exceptional Memory Fast!" These are typical examples of a number of advertising slogans for apps, books, pills, and programs. Memory, however, is complex, not fully understood, and requires intensive focus and understanding. Long-term memory and habit formation take time and hard work to develop—there is no quick fix or simple solution when it comes to building memory.

Unfortunately, commercial, computer-based memory training programs are based on this neurocentric approach. These programs claim to benefit those suffering from purported ADHD, dyslexia, language disorders, poor academic performance, the dementias, mental ill-health, and many other issues. Some claim to even boost IQ or EQ scores.[16] These programs are used around the world in educational institutions and clinics, and most are digital platforms that involve tasks in which participants are given memory tests designed to be challenging.

However, research shows that the short-term memory and sensory skills developed in these so-called brain games do not necessarily develop deep thinking or meaningful cognitive skills that change behavior in ways that lead to success.[17] These games do not improve the kind of intelligence that helps people intellectualize, reason, solve problems, or make wise choices. In contrast, mental training via deep thinking and understanding to build memory and learn—as put forward in my techniques in this book—increases the numbers of neurons that *survive*, particularly when the training goals are challenging.[18] This survival of neurons with their dendrites (where memory is actually stored) means long-term, useful, and meaningful memories are formed.

In fact, according to a study published by the American Psychological Association (APA), working memory training from these brain games is unlikely to be an effective treatment for children suffering from learning disorders.[19] Likewise, memory training tasks appear to have limited effect on healthy adults and children looking to do better in school or improve their intellectual and cognitive skills.[20]

Many programs bring rote memory more into play than comprehension—at their peril. We are not designed to remember everything and anything. We are designed to remember what we *need* to succeed. This requires comprehension and deep, focused understanding. We need to learn *what* to learn and *how* to learn.

I will explain how to build meaningful memories in chapter 20, memories that not only increase intelligence but enhance brain health and reflect the complexity of the thinking process.[21] There are a great number of helpful techniques to improve memory, but they act on a particular type of memory only, whether it is mnemonics, repetitions of the same stimulus, and so on. I prefer to focus on teaching you how to build memory that is *useful*, significant, and able to help you succeed and thrive in school, the workplace, and life. Like my patients, once you learn how to learn using your mind, you will notice a significant increase in your ability to resolve problems and improve cognitive flexibility in *addition* to building meaningful memory.

A growing body of evidence shows how our thought lives have incredible power over our intellectual, emotional, cognitive, and physical well-being. Our thoughts can either limit us to what we believe we can do or free us to develop abilities well beyond our expectations or the expectations of others. When we choose a mindset that extends our abilities rather than limits them, we will experience greater intellectual satisfaction, emotional control, and mental and physical health.

But how do we do this? How can we harness the power of our thoughts to think deeply, learn powerfully, and deal with the problems of the fast-paced digital age in order to lead lives filled with meaning? How do we achieve success? For over three decades, I have worked with thousands of families, children, teenagers, and adults diagnosed with ADHD, autism, dementias, and other learning and emotional difficulties, teaching them how to resolve their challenges and improve their thinking. My experience, both professionally and personally, as well as the testimonies from individuals who have watched my TV shows[22] and read my other books, reveal that, if you teach people how to think deeply, they can do anything they put their minds to. They can learn *how* to learn.

Regardless of what anyone has told you, you can learn. You can succeed at life. When you learn how to learn, exploring, understanding, and mastering the art of mental self-care, you can go beyond mindfulness, developing a whole mind lifestyle that allows you to transform your neighborhood, your community, your nation, and your world.

SECTION ONE

The Mindset Guide

ONE

Thinking and Learning to Succeed

A mindset is an attitude, or a cluster of thoughts with attached information and emotions that generate a particular perception. They shape how you see and interact with the world. They can catapult you forward, allowing you to achieve your dreams, or put you in reverse drive if you are not careful. A mindset is therefore a significant mental resource and source of power. Your mindsets set your expectation levels, which will either be positive or negative.

Every moment of every day, your brain and body are physically reacting and changing in response to the thoughts that run through your mind—your mindsets add "flavor" to your thoughts, making your brain and body work for you or against you. And because you control your mindsets—they are not some preprogrammed function—it's you that is actually making your brain and body work for you. Understanding how mindsets form and how they change your thinking is a practical and helpful way to understand the power of your mind to change your brain. Mindsets help you see the power of your perceptions while optimizing your thought life by generating the correct perceptions, revealing your inner strength and resilience. The correct mindsets are integral to succeeding in school, work, and life.

Your brain responds to your life choices—which are influenced by your mindsets. You are not controlled by your biology, no matter how emotionally flat or chaotic your mind feels at any given moment in time.[1] Just *thinking* about something can cause your brain to change through the waves of energy that are generated, on a structural level through genetic expression and on a chemical level through the release of neurotransmitters. The power of the mind to change the brain is incredibly exciting and hopeful!

Our thoughts can improve our peace, health, vision, fitness, strength, and much more.[2] The ability to think, feel, and choose and build thoughts into mindsets is one of the most powerful things in the universe, because this power is the source of all human creativity and imagination. As scientist Lynne McTaggart notes, "a thought is not only a thing; a thought is a thing that influences other things."[3] Where your mind goes, your life follows.

Research, as well as common sense, shows that believing you will succeed is a precursor to success.[4] Conversely, thinking that you are limited is itself a limiting factor—a nocebo effect.[5] We can *choose* to adopt a mindset that improves our creativity and functionality in general, or we can choose to adopt an attitude that constrains us.

The truth is, we don't have to learn to think outside the box. We have to recognize that the "box" is a figment of our imagination— we are as intelligent as we want to be. The purpose of this book is to help you discover how unlimited your ability to think truly is. You *can* design and sculpt your brain with your thoughts.

What Happens When You Think

Think of your mind as the movement of information as energy through your nervous system. Each thought has quantum energy and electrochemical and electromagnetic signals, which flow throughout your brain and body largely below the level of awareness in your nonconscious mind (see chapter 21 for more on this). Just thinking about a loved one, for example, can cause positive structural changes in the caudate nucleus of the brain, which is closely linked to feelings of reward and happiness.[6] Likewise, healthy electromagnetic signals and quantum fields fire up across the entire brain and body in response to a good attitude, giving you strength to face the day.[7]

The converse also applies. Stress, which is actually good for you, can become incredibly toxic, depending on your perception of the situation.[8] The other day, a friend was telling me how just driving past her previous workplace brought back significant physical heart pain, which she used to experience daily in the toxic work environment. While still there, this friend was considering seeing a cardiac specialist due to the severity of her toxic stress-related symptoms, but they disappeared once she resigned. The treatment in this case wasn't medication or potential surgery, it was the mental self-care decision to get another job!

Research in quantum physics and the mind-body connection shows the signals of the mind, which are considered nonphysical light waves or packets of energy, form 90 to 99 percent of who we are. These waves are our dominant reality; we cannot ignore the intangible, powerful mind element of who we are as humans.[9] As thoughts travel through our brains at quantum speeds, neurons fire together in distinctive ways based on the specific information being handled, and those patterns of neural activity transform our neural structure (you will learn more about this in chapter 22). Essentially, the way you think, through the mindsets you adopt, will influence the neural correlates in your brain, thereby influencing your words and actions. In turn, these words and actions influence the brain, and a feedback loop is established based on this mindset. A feedback loop can be changed any time you desire through your *choice* to change your mindset. An interesting study, for example, indicated that instead of trying to *calm down* to cope with preperformance anxiety such as meeting with a boss, public speaking, or writing a math exam, reconceptualizing the anxiety as *excitement* while taking deep slow breaths (which dissipates cortisol) helped people cope better. Choosing to shift from a threat mindset to an opportunity mindset changes functioning.[10]

You have so much power in you to thrive instead of strive. When people consciously choose to practice operating in a mindset of gratitude, for instance, they get a surge of rewarding neurotransmitters such as dopamine and experience a general sense of being alert and a brightening of the mind. The path to success starts with our thinking, and our brain will respond accordingly.

If, however, you bombard the 75 to 100 trillion cells of your brain and body with toxic signals from negative thoughts, you negatively influence the quantum actions and genetic expression in your cells, *training* them to reproduce negativity in the future. Thinking in this way, you develop a negative mindset that can wreak havoc in your mind, brain, and body. These negative mindsets are not, however, your destiny. You can change any mindset by transforming the way you think, feel, and choose. You can choose to bombard the cells of your body with positivity, honing in on your natural proclivity toward love.[11] We are wired with an optimism bias.

As long as you can breathe, your brain can make new neurons in a process called neurogenesis.[12] Stem cells persist in the adult brain and generate new neurons throughout life; thousands of new cells are created on a daily basis. These thousands of new neurons that are added into the brain each day do not survive. However, one of the most effective ways to keep these cells from dying (which increases toxic levels in your brain and body) is by thinking and learning properly.[13] This is exactly what I will be teaching you to do in section 3 of this book with the Switch On Your Brain 5-Step Learning Process. Different signals promote stem cells to form neurons that migrate to their place of action.[14] You also have glial cells in your brain that produce more cells on a daily basis.[15] These cells are essentially "housekeepers" and are also involved in cognition.

In fact, you have the power to change toxic mindsets with your customized thinking about every ten seconds! Your brain is finely attuned to your mind; it is designed to respond to your conscious thinking (see chapter 21).

This is truly what it means to renew and redesign your mind and bring all rogue thoughts into captivity. This also means you *can* redesign your brain with your mindset by choosing to be more optimistic and adopting healthy thinking practices such as the mental self-care techniques you will learn about in this book. This process of reappraising and realigning your mindsets back to your natural wired-for-love design is integral to the life well-lived. It is a way of deliberately and intentionally paying attention to what you think, say, and do in a self-reflective and self-regulatory way. And it all hinges on what you *choose* to think about.

Genetic Expression and Mindful Thinking

Your thinking, feeling, and choosing impacts your genetic expression. You switch genes on and off with every thought you have, and every thought you have is a response to the way you *see* and perceive your life experiences.[16] Research actually shows that only about 5 percent of genetic mutations directly cause health issues.[17] Roughly 95 percent of genes are influenced by life factors and lifestyle choices.[18] Your genetic activity is largely determined by your thoughts, attitudes, and perceptions, which collectively form your mindset.

So how do you control your genetic expression? The science of epigenetics shows us that our thoughts control our biology,[19] and perceptions are made of our thoughts, which create our mindsets. Our lifestyle choices can actually be traced to the genetic level. What you are thinking at any one moment becomes vitally important because your thoughts determine the signals your genes receive. By changing your thoughts, you change your mindsets, and, in turn, you can influence and shape your own genetic readout. Research even shows that your mindsets can impact how you age![20]

The more you learn to think in your unique and powerful customized way, which you will read about in section 2, the more mindful, self-reflective, and self-regulating you will become in your thinking; you will develop successful mindsets. The healthier the input signal, the healthier the output of your genetic expression, and the healthier and more successful you will be.

I cannot stress enough the power of learning to control and activate the power of mindsets to influence life outcomes. During my academic research and in my clinical practice, I observed over and over again just how extremely important positive mental self-care was in succeeding versus surviving, because of the impact of thinking on our memory and our mental and physical health.

Of course, we are all different. We all think differently, and how we think differently influences the effectiveness of building useful, sustainable memory. And when we learn how *we*, as unique individuals, think and learn, we have a sense of purpose, which according to recent research increases the tendency to healthier living and therefore longevity. Thus, through thinking in our wired-for-love mode,[21] partnered with healthy eating, sleeping, and exercising habits,[22] we can develop deep-rooted memories while reducing the risk of mental ill-health, educational problems, and degenerative diseases. Strong evidence is available suggesting controlling one's inner thought life and detoxing the mind is a preventative against Alzheimer's.[23] This is real mental self-care that leads to success. (For more on detoxing the mind, see my app at drleaf.com.)

Understanding your "gift," your customized thinking, and how to use the Switch On Your Brain 5-Step Learning Process will activate and sustain the power of positive mindsets, which, in turn, will give you direct access to influencing your genetic activity in a beneficial way. As you begin to understand and realize how much power you have in your mind, you will start using your thoughts to work *for* you instead of *against* you.

Wired for Love

We are wired to think positively with optimism.[24] Your body and brain are finely attuned to your uniqueness and the positivity of your mind. You are essentially wired for love, right down to the genetic level; the more you improve your mental self-care habits, the more your brain and body will respond in positive ways.[25]

Yet, when you have a negative mindset, which is out of sync with your wired-for-love design, you damage the brain and body. You begin to function at a compromised level, which affects your mental and physical health. Fortunately, you can combat this negative spiral when you choose to change your mindset, healing the damage and improving the way you function. You can rewrite the story of your past![26]

Cultivating healthy, successful mindsets is the key ingredient to achieving a thriving lifestyle. We all have significant internal resources to think, learn, and succeed at life, but these often go unused or are misused. Through the knowledge you gain from this book, you will learn how to harness the power of your mind for success.

However, before we explore what these successful mindsets look like, we have to first understand what it means to be "wired for love." There isn't a structure, tissue, cell, protein, molecule, atom, or quantum wave that is designed for toxic thinking; we are wired for love and we learn to fear.[27]

Does that mean that all types of fear are inherently bad? Not necessarily. We love life, for example, so we fear things that can take life away from us, and thus we avoid these things, such as running in front of a moving car or traveling through dangerous areas late at night. Similarly, we experience grief because we love. *Love* is an umbrella term for all the characteristics we value as human beings, such as gratitude, joy, peace, patience, kindness, positivity, happiness, and so on. I therefore use "love mindsets" to refer to all types of mindsets that help us prosper as we go about our daily activities. When we operate in love-based mindsets, we enhance our brain, body, mind, and spiritual health.[28] Love is about succeeding, not merely surviving. A life of love is "the good life."

Fear, on the other hand, is distorted love. It is the opposite of love, just as ingratitude is the opposite of gratitude and cruelty is the opposite of kindness. Fear eats away at us, crippling our ability to live the kind of life we want to live. A fearful mindset focuses on the absence of love; the fear of failure, for example, stifles creativity and the imagination, hindering an individual's ability to pursue his or her goals and dreams.

Our mindsets set the tone for how we approach the events and circumstances of life, which are often out of our control. We are designed to react in a love mindset, which doesn't always mean things are going to be easy but does mean we can shift into success mode and manage a situation more effectively.

Brain plasticity means the changes that occur in the brain as a result of thinking and lifestyle choices. Brain plasticity allows us to master simple skills or sports and also allows us to train ourselves to be more positive, whether it is raining or the sun is shining, literally and figuratively. I did some of the first neuroplasticity research back in the eighties, showing how intentional, deliberate thinking changes intellectual, cognitive, emotional, social, and academic performance.[29] In my practical clinical experience, the power of neuroplasticity continued to play out with the people I worked with—you can change your brain with your mind, and, by doing so, change your life.

We *can* retrain the brain to focus on the good things in life. We step into our "normal" when we do this, because we are wired for love. Having an "attitude of gratitude," so to speak, enables us to see more possibilities, to feel more energy, and to succeed at higher levels in our lives.

I emphasize *retraining* the brain as opposed to training the brain. It is incorrect to assume that the brain has a negative bias and that we have to fight off the brain's natural tendency to scan for and spot the undesirable. This kind of negative mindset will actually work against the natural optimism bias of brain function and upset thinking patterns!

As I mentioned above, the brain is wired for the positive, which is also called the optimism bias, or what I call the *wired-for-love bias*. Occasionally, you may feel like the negative dominates your life, but take a moment to analyze your thoughts. What do you think about the most? Whatever you think about the most will grow; if you are thinking about something daily, within approximately two months your brain has changed to accommodate this pattern of thought (see more on this in chapter 21, on memory). You plant these thoughts deep into your nonconscious mind, allowing them free rein to shape your mindset, which in turn affects your future thoughts, words, and actions. We merge with our environments; whatever we think about the most will have the most energy and will dominate our thinking, the good and the bad. In section 3 of this book I show how this happens, and how just seven minutes a day of directed, intentional thinking for sixty three days can renew your thinking!

Indeed, we can harness the brain's plasticity by using our mind to train our brain to build normal positive patterns. This is called *automatization* and involves the reconceptualization of memory—that is the deliberate, intentional, mindful, and intellectual redesigning of thoughts (and thus the structure of the brain) over time.

Automatization is not incredibly difficult, but it does require time, discipline, and effort. If asked, I am certain you would be able to point out your positive and negative thinking habits, your love and fear mindsets. You have already been practicing building mindsets, albeit without consciously knowing the technique! The conscious control of this process can take you to a whole new level of life, allowing you to function successfully on both a personal and professional level. You will learn to develop not only a positive outlook but also a sense of mastery and intellectual satisfaction that allows you to be more creative. It's time to start harnessing your powerful mind to change your life!

TWO

The Thinker Mindset

It is easy in today's age to have access to any number of readily available stimuli. Social media, email, texting, ebooks, Facetime, Skype, chat rooms—you name it, you literally have a world of data at your fingertips. According to the American Psychological Association's Stress in America Survey 2017, between 2005 and 2015, the percentage of adults using social media skyrocketed from 7 percent to 65 percent. In young adults ages eighteen to twenty-nine, that usage increased from 12 percent to 90 percent in that same time period.[1]

You may be so connected that you have forgotten how to spend time just being alone with your thoughts. When was the last time you struck the pose—figuratively speaking—of the sculptor Auguste Rodin's famous statue *The Thinker*? Do you fear being alone with yourself? Can you be alone with yourself? Just you and your thoughts?

The need to be constantly occupied does not just concern "kids these days." One recent study found that being alone with one's thoughts is considered an unpleasant experience by the majority of people of *all* ages.[2] In a series of eleven studies done by

Timothy Wilson and colleagues at the University of Virginia and Harvard, a number of the participants of all age ranges (eighteen to seventy-seven years) battled spending six to fifteen minutes alone with nothing to do but think, daydream, and ponder. The majority of the participants didn't enjoy being alone with their thoughts, while some preferred even shocking themselves to sitting and thinking! The conclusions of this study indicate that most of the participants preferred to be doing something, even something negative, rather than just using their imagination for several minutes.

Indeed, more and more of us, of all ages, prefer aimlessly scrolling through Instagram, Facebook, online shopping apps, or random things on our devices than just sitting and thinking. Although we are more connected, literally, we are more isolated than ever before. Surveys have actually found that spending more time on social media and other "screen" activities correlates strongly with lower levels of happiness, higher feelings of loneliness and depression, and a greater risk of suicide.[3]

Jean Twenge, who has been researching generational differences for the past three decades, says that the impact of these devices has not yet been fully recognized or understood.[4] Looking at the impact of increased phone usage, much of the harm of social media can be attributed to what the internet terms "FOMO," or fear of missing out on the fun everyone else seems to be having.[5] Twenge acknowledges the positive side of technology, which has led to increased confidence, open-mindedness, and ambition, but also understands that the technological revolution has a dark side, with increasing cynicism, loneliness, anxiousness, and depression plaguing the modern mind. The correlations between mental ill-health, loneliness, isolation, and smartphone use are strong enough to suggest that we should not only ask our children to put down the phone but ourselves as well.

Of course, in every generation what it means to be an individual in society changes, sometimes dramatically. Yet the ability to think about, process, and maintain a balanced lifestyle is always a top priority when it comes to coping with social change, and "thinker" moments are an integral part of our mental self-care regimen. The brain needs "thinker" time for its health and functioning, including the prevention of dementias!

Remember, the brain is neuroplastic—it is constantly changing. We merge with our environments through our choices, including how long we decide to spend on our phone. "Thinker" time is very important, because it balances our minds, allowing us to observe our environment before we just let it influence and direct our thinking.

We need downtime to function optimally. To cope with the demands of life, our minds and brains need to internally "reboot," which can only happen when we are alone with our thoughts. We literally need to switch off all external stimuli, giving our thoughts some quality "me time."

Contrary to popular belief, the mind does not grind to a halt when you are doing nothing. Spontaneous thought processes, including mind-wandering, creative thinking, and daydreaming, arise when thoughts are relatively free from focused thinking and external influences. This type of *internal* thinking actually plays an important role in contributing to the richness of *intentional* thinking and subsequent learning, adding a powerful creative aspect to our lives. Learning in the "thinker" moments can enhance our success in work, school, and life. Without this spontaneous thinking mode, we wouldn't be able to reach those insights and inspirational highs that change our world. Like Isaac Newton, we should all spend more time sitting under trees and just thinking!

"Thinker" moments actually increase and develop our intelligence and the efficiency of our thinking. A 2017 study from the Georgia Institute of Technology suggests that daydreaming during meetings or school, for example, indicates that someone is smart and creative.[6] Someone who can daydream can zone out of conversations or tasks, when appropriate, then naturally tune back in without missing important points or steps.[7] The "absent-minded professor" off in their own world, sometimes oblivious to surroundings, or the student or work colleague who checks out mentally and looks away for a few moments to daydream, are actually developing their mind and are often thinking deeply about the matter at hand.

A University of British Columbia–led review of mind-wandering research highlights the importance of allowing our mind to just think.[8] Lead researcher Kalina Christoff notes that thoughts can sometimes move freely and, at other times, can keep coming back to the same concept or idea, getting stuck in the rumination process.[9] In my experience, helping my patients analyze and write down their thoughts in a self-reflective way, in those "thinker" moments when they were potentially ruminating and getting stuck, was an effective way to develop their imagination. I would help them work out which thoughts were free flowing and track their direction over time, as well as noting which thoughts were getting stuck. My patients found it especially helpful to then evaluate whether these thoughts were giving them a sense of peace or making them concerned, and then to look for an alternate way of thinking to reconceptualize the disturbing thought or thoughts. I would then teach them to practice developing the newly reconceptualized positive thoughts, automatizing them over time into helpful, useful, and successful memories. I will describe this process in greater detail in chapter 20.

The process of understanding what allows free thinking, and what allows something to get "stuck in our heads," is crucial to mental self-care. Analyzing our thoughts in this way gives insight into how we can actually capture and change toxic and intrusive thoughts that are blocking our success.

The mind-wandering "thinker" state can be highjacked, so to speak, by existing toxic thoughts moving up from our nonconscious mind, unless we control them.[10] Deliberate, negative thinking like *I can't do it* or *This is too hard* can also poison our "thinker" moments, which can result in mental and physical damage in the brain and body, setting the stage for future mind and brain issues, including the dementias, which are largely preventable. These types of thoughts can literally paralyze our imagination, inhibiting success in school, life, and work, and create negative reinforcing feedback loops. It is thus incredibly important to our present and future to have "thinker" moments that allow us to control our thoughts, using them to our advantage.

Controlling the mind-wandering "thinker" is known as an *awake resting state*.[11] It activates the coexisting default mode network (DMN) and task positive network (TPN) in the brain in a constructive and healthy way.[12] These networks form the brain's inner life with the DMN dominating and becoming especially active when the mind is introspective and thinking deeply in a directed rest or idling state. The DMN is a primary network that we switch into when we switch off from the outside world and move into a state of focused mindfulness. It activates to even higher levels when a person is daydreaming, introspecting, or letting his or her mind wander in an organized exploratory way through the endless myriad of thoughts within the deep spiritual nonconscious part of who we are. The TPN, on the other hand, supports the active thinking required for making decisions. So, as we focus our thinking and activate the DMN, at some point in our thinking process we move into active decision making. This activates the TPN, and we experience this as action.[13] Recent research confirms how important working on our inner lives, using the DMN, is in decreasing the incidence of Alzheimer's disease.[14] The DMN is known to be implicated in the pathological process of the disease.

Being alone with our thoughts can also provide valuable and potent insight into how we function[15] and can positively influence our judgment and decisions.[16] As Socrates once said, "the unexamined life is not worth living." Thinker moments allow us to examine our own internal lives and develop our unique imagination.[17]

Research from Concordia University and fifteen other universities worldwide shows that 94 percent of people examined across six continents experience unwanted, intrusive thoughts, images, and/or impulses.[18] The team of researchers found that the thoughts, images, and impulses symptomatic of obsessive compulsive disorder (OCD) are actually *widespread globally*, and that this study shows it's not the unwanted, intrusive thoughts that are the problem but the way they are *managed*.[19] The OCD label is thus a description of how a person manages traumatic experiences through their thinking rather than a disease that destroys someone's life.[20]

Management of thoughts is the key to success, which is why it is the overriding objective of all my work, research, books, and programs. It is your perceptions of your thoughts, and what you do with your thoughts, that are important. Learning to capture thoughts and evaluate them logically by developing a thinker mindset is one of the most significant parts of any mental self-care regimen, allowing us to become more self-evaluative and self-regulatory. To this end, we should take the poem "Leisure" by William Davies to heart:

> What is this life if, full of care,
> We have no time to stand and stare.
> No time to stand beneath the boughs
> And stare as long as sheep or cows.
> No time to see, when woods we pass,
> Where squirrels hide their nuts in grass.
> No time to see, in broad daylight,
> Streams full of stars, like skies at night.
> No time to turn at Beauty's glance,
> And watch her feet, how they can dance.
> No time to wait till her mouth can
> Enrich that smile her eyes began.
> A poor life this if, full of care,
> We have no time to stand and stare.[21]

Thinker Mindset Activation Tips

1. Are cellphones and other devices stealing your "thinker" moments? Observe yourself for several days, making note of how much you use technology and if this is happening to you.

2. The average person spends up to eight hours a day using technology. Some of the worst effects of electronic devices seem to be mitigated when devices are used less than two hours a day.[22] Find ways to limit your use of technology throughout the day.

3. Thinker moments aren't an odd quirk of the mind but are natural and spontaneous. Allocate time, at least sixteen minutes a day, to just thinking and allowing your mind to wander. You can spread this across the day in two or three intervals.

4. Thinker moments actually increase and develop our intelligence and mind and brain efficiency. When you don't feel like being a "thinker," remember that these moments increase your intelligence!

5. Thinker moments are preventative against dementias because they enhance brain health. When you don't feel like being a "thinker," remember that these moments increase your brain health and help prevent dementia!

6. Thinker moments teach you how to live the self-examined life. As your mind wanders, think about what you are thinking and your own experiences, perhaps writing about your thoughts in a journal or notepad.

7. During your thinker moments, write down, in a self-reflective way, which thoughts are free-flowing as well as which thoughts get stuck. Track the direction of free-flowing thoughts over time. Capture and change the thoughts that get stuck. (See chapter 20 for more details on how to do this.)

8. Evaluate whether your thoughts give you a sense of peace or make you worried. If your thoughts concern you, think

differently about the same thing every time that thought pops up. In other words, reconceptualize the disturbing thought.

9. Practice developing the newly reconceptualized positive thought daily and automatizing it over time into helpful, useful, and successful memory. (See chapter 20 for more details on how to do this and my app on how to detox your thoughts at drleaf.com or your app store.)

THREE

The Controlled
Thinking Mindset

How many could-have, would-have or should-have statements have you uttered today? How many if-onlys? How many times have you replayed a bad conversation or situation in your head, thinking about how it could have gone differently? How many times have you thought of what may happen in the future, worrying about something you cannot control? How much time do you spend speculating? Do thoughts just run through your brain, and you feel like you cannot control them? Are you honest with yourself, or do you run from your thoughts and feelings? Do you go through the motions of the day, not really committed to a goal, saying one thing but meaning another? Is your thinking distorted? Have you formed a personal identity around a problem or disease you are facing? Do you speak about "my arthritis," "my multiple sclerosis," or "my heart problem"? Do you ever make comments like "Nothing ever goes right for me," "Everything I touch fails," or "I always mess up"? Does your mind often feel foggy? Do you battle with remembering things? Do you battle to learn?

If you answered yes to any one of these questions, you are being human in a world full of challenges! We all face challenges in life, and we all need to learn how to consciously control our thought lives, every moment of every day, to cope and not break. This is why it's so important to understand the creative power of our ability to choose. Mind-body research increasingly points to the fact that consciously controlling your thoughts is one of the best ways, if not the *best* way, of detoxing your brain and body. Learning how to renew the mind enables you to get rid of toxic thoughts and emotions that block success.

Let us look at something many experience, especially with age: back pain. Dr. John Sarno, a professor of clinical rehabilitation medicine at New York University and an author, proposes that most back pain stems from psychological rather than physiological problems.[1] Sarno notes how our thoughts can heal or harm the body. In the latter case, toxic thoughts can potentially cause debilitating back pain in specific circumstances.

Consciously controlling your thought life means that you do not allow thoughts to rampage through your mind. Instead, you learn to engage interactively with each thought, taking control over and learning to enjoy the moment you are in. Essentially, your job is to analyze a thought before you decide either to accept or reject it.

Controlling your thoughts sounds great, but how do you do it? You start by "looking" at your mental processes. And no, you do not crack open your skull like an egg and have a look at what is going on inside your brain! It is possible, however, to learn about your mental processes through thinking about your thinking and choosing what to think about.[2] This process of self-reflection is not only possible, it's essential.

Toxic thoughts come in many guises. On the surface, thoughts like *I must do well* or *I must finish this in the next thirty minutes* seem all right, but when you look at them closely and analyze the feelings they generate, you will see how these thoughts may not be serving you well. Demanding unrealistic performance from yourself and others, for instance, puts your mind and body into toxic stress mode, which has a negative effect on your brain and body health.[3] This type of pressure can also lead to haphazard, distracted thinking, which certainly doesn't help matters!

If you don't train yourself to control your thought life, you may end up thinking more toxic thoughts and generating more toxic emotions. These negative thought patterns can inhibit your ability to think clearly, understand, and learn—they are roadblocks on the road to success. This type of thinking can also allow other illnesses and diseases to take root.

It is important to remember that thoughts create your mood and influence how you feel physically. When you experience a fear-based emotion, you will feel "under the weather" and your thoughts will be shaped by your negativity. Your thoughts will become distorted and you will lose the joy of the "now" moment.

To control your thought life, you have to activate and continually make use of the quantum principle of *superposition*, which is the ability to focus on incoming information and on upcoming memories from your nonconscious mind. As you think about these thoughts, you need to analyze them in as objective a way as possible before you choose which to believe and which to reject.[4]

But what does superposition look like? Imagine yourself sitting on a surfboard and a "magic breeze" is blowing through the networks of your mind as you are thinking, feeling, and choosing which way you want to tip the surfboard: either to ride the wave or to fall back and wait for the next wave. It's as though time has frozen for a moment. This breeze makes you aware of some memories related to the current situation and your thinking patterns, preparing your brain to build a new memory. If you ask, answer, and discuss while in superposition (while on the surfboard), you are in effect "capturing thoughts." It is almost as if you are watching yourself, becoming aware of what you are thinking, feeling, and focusing on in as much detail as you can in the now moment—that is, in the present. I call this the Multiple

Perspective Advantage, or MPA for short (I have written on this extensively in my other books and online programs and app on how to detox your mind at drleaf.com).[5] When you consciously engage with information that is coming into your brain in this way, you will be able to instinctively select around 15 to 35 percent of what you read, hear, and see, while getting rid of the remaining 65 to 85 percent that is superfluous and can have a negative effect on your ability to focus and build memory. When you use your MPA, your senses will finely tune in to the detail of the now moment—an enriching experience that will help you feel happier and more at peace.

Mindfulness allows you to develop a heightened sense of awareness in the present moment, accepting things as they are without judgment and emotional reactivity. When you step into superposition and use your MPA, you go *beyond mindfulness*. In this objective state, you are capturing and reconceptualizing toxic and chaotic thoughts and building healthy, organized thoughts. This second step is necessary to stabilize attention and develop thinking habits that you will actually use in your life.

A "controlled thinking" mindset helps you to intentionally shift your focus. It allows you to determine your own performance, rather than getting stuck replaying negative experiences in your head.

Indeed, much research, including my own,[6] consistently shows that if you do not capture thoughts and monitor incoming information, it is hard to change toxic and chaotic thoughts, which will steal your mental peace and your ability to build useful memory and learn. As humans, we are designed to engage with information; we are designed to build our brains.

Talking to yourself out loud can help you control your thinking, even if it's just a whisper. In fact, talking out loud enhances your ability to think by stimulating the corpus callosum (which joins the two hemispheres of the brain) to function at a much higher level.[7] It also provides extra auditory stimulation to enhance the now-moment experience, and is an excellent way of looking at your thoughts and the feelings they generate before you decide whether or not they deserve to be discarded as toxic or retained as beneficial.

Never let thoughts just wander through your mind unchecked. If thoughts are toxic, they can affect your ability to build healthy memories and make you ill. We should never forget that thoughts are real things—they impact brain and body functionality, thereby impacting your quality of life. Toxic stress has even been shown to reduce the size of certain structures in the brain![8]

As discussed in chapter 2, daydreaming and mind wandering can be good for you. These moments only become a problem when they are chaotic and unmanaged, because the chaos stops you from benefitting from and enjoying your thoughts. For example, ruminating on the past in a negative way, obsessing on an issue or desire, or shifting crazily and haphazardly between thoughts will steal the joy of the now moment. You need to use thinker moments for and not against yourself through learning to control your thoughts.

When you use your mind to consciously take control of your thought life, you will find that it does not take long to see the benefits. Studies show that a positive thinking environment can lead to significant structural changes in the brain's cortex in just four days.[9] Frequent, positive, and challenging learning experiences increase intelligence in a relatively short amount of time.[10] My own research demonstrates that learning potential can be increased 35 to 75 percent if people are taught how to understand the mind-brain/body connection, and to deliberately think in ways that encourage learning and memory formation.[11] Detoxing the brain by controlling your thought life won't only make you feel better but will also make you smarter.

Cutting-edge brain research over the past few decades shows that intelligence is not static; it can be enhanced or reduced by what you decide to think about. You control your brain by your thought life—you can make yourself healthier and smarter. In my clinical practice, several of my patients increased their IQ from average to genius, even if their brains were injured![12]

Five to seven memories move into our conscious awareness every few moments. We need to make sure we use these memories to help us understand the incoming thoughts from our environments and not to distract us. We are essentially training ourselves to focus and pay more attention as we "do life."

Leonardo da Vinci purportedly said, "An average human looks without seeing, listens without hearing, touches without feeling, eats without tasting, moves without physical awareness, inhales without awareness of odor or fragrance, and talks without thinking."[13] We need to learn to savor the pleasure of now and not just marinate in the misery of the past or imagine that the grass will be greener in the future. When we choose to truly tune in to the now—to see, listen, feel, move, taste, and inhale the present, using all our senses to soak up the minute beauty of the moment—we enhance our thinking and thereby enhance our ability to learn and succeed at life.

Controlled Thinking Mindset Activation Tips

1. Never let thoughts just wander through your mind unchecked. Focus on the now moment and observe your thoughts and feelings.

2. Using superposition, analyze a thought before you decide either to accept or reject it.

3. Analytically ask, answer, and discuss while in superposition, "capturing those thoughts." (See chapter 20 for full details on how to do this.)

4. When you consciously engage with information that is coming into your brain and think about it purposefully, select approximately 15 to 35 percent of what you read, hear, and see.

5. Reconceptualize (redesign) thoughts that are holding you
   back by deciding what thought you would rather have and
   then work toward eliminating the toxic thought and building
   something better. Here is an example:

   Start with acknowledging and articulating thoughts weigh-
   ing you down—ones that don't serve any useful purpose beyond
   keeping you stuck. Now ask yourself questions rather than
   issuing commands to yourself—this is a much more effective
   way to reconceptualize because it opens up exploration, creates
   possibility, and distances you from what you are thinking, giving
   you a safe space for change. You can also label your emotions
   in a nonjudgmental way to give yourself some distance from
   them in order to deal with them.

   (See chapter 21 for more information on the time frame
   involved, and see www.21daybraindetox.com for an online
   program on how to do this as well as my app on how to detox
   your thoughts at drleaf.com or your app store.)

FOUR

The Words Mindset

No discussion of thoughts and their impact on your health would be complete without examining words, the fruit of your thoughts. The words you speak are electromagnetic and quantum life forces that come from thoughts inside your brain, which you build into your mind by thinking, feeling, and choosing over time.[1] These words contain power and *reflect* your thought life, influencing the world around you and the circumstances of your life. Your words are therefore very useful, since they provide insight into what is holding you back or propelling you forward.

The words you speak feed back into the physical thoughts you have built into your mind, reinforcing the memory they came from. When you make negative statements, you release negative chemicals. These chemicals allow negative memories to grow stronger, especially if you continue to allow these thoughts to dominate your thinking. Whatever you think about the most grows. When you constantly think about something negative and speak about it, it can become a negative stronghold that controls your attitude and life. Every time you utter a negative statement, you release negative quantum energy and upset the balance of peptides, which affects the environment of the brain and puts the body into toxic stress.[2]

On the other hand, the more you speak positively, the more you think positively! Please note, I am talking about *much more* than just positive thinking or positive affirmations, because framing your world with words is not just about talking positively. The problem with positive affirmations, per se, is that they operate at the surface level of conscious thinking but do not align with the nonconscious mind where limiting beliefs really reside (see section 4).

Your words have to be backed up with honesty and integrity, or what in psychological terms is called *cognitive congruence*. Positive affirmations only work when you believe what you say. If you lie to yourself, you will experience *cognitive dissonance*, the opposite of cognitive congruence, which can impact your mental and physical health because you are creating an internal war. Whitewashing your toxic thoughts and words with positive-thinking affirmations is merely a temporary fix, a band-aid approach.

What you do and say on the outside must reflect what you think and *actually believe* on the inside. The root (what you really are thinking) and the fruit (what you are saying) need to match up, or you are going to create neurochemical chaos in the brain. A lack of congruence causes toxic stress and affects the way information is processed and memory is built. Being more intentionally mindful about what you want to say, what you are saying, and what you are actually thinking about what you are saying bring all sorts of prefrontal resources to help get the amygdala unstuck from toxic emotions. This happens because the more intentionally mindful you are, the more activation you have in the right ventrolateral prefrontal cortex and the less activation you have in the amygdala in response—and this is a good thing![3]

For example, using a positive affirmation like "I am brilliant and successful" may backfire if you don't *truly, deeply* believe it at the nonconscious level. To effectively reconceptualize your thinking and your resultant words, rather, consider who you are *becoming*, focusing on your progress. A more realistic positive statement would be something like "I believe I have the potential to release the brilliance inside of me, and each day I will spend one to three minutes consciously and deliberately working toward achieving this goal." So you put a positive spin onto the honest reality of what you are feeling in the now moment. You redesign your future, because your future is in your hands. The love and support of those we trust is integral to this process, but ultimately *you* have to make the choice to change and move forward.

Framing your world with your words, therefore, involves replacing negative thinking and words by changing your word mindset. When you start speaking positive words, words that are rooted in honest thinking, you literally destroy the old toxic memory and grow a beautiful new memory to replace the painful and oppressive one. Of course, you will still remember what happened to you in the past, but the memory has been reconceptualized—it no longer rules your life. Instead it becomes a rich part of your character.

Congruent thinking, not positive words, creates the necessary changes in the brain. This type of thinking takes time and effort, because you have to be aware of your words and the mindset behind them. This awareness enables you to capture these thoughts and change them. You cannot fix a problem you do not even acknowledge is there, after all. You cannot fix a problem in an instant, either. Success comes from the realization that we do not always measure up to our dreams. Often we have to change our direction or acknowledge we are evolving as we are heading to get where we want to go. And this takes time, so give yourself the necessary space to do this.

Words Mindset Activation Tips

1. Acknowledge that an issue exists through observing the words you are speaking and the impact they have on you and on other people and things in your life. Become intentionally mindful about this.

2. Examine your words and compare them to the thoughts they came from. Are they congruent? If not, write down the two and start working toward congruency over cycles of twenty-one days. (See chapter 20 for more on this.)

3. Practice going into superposition and taking time to examine your words, thinking about what is wrong, or what is right, with what you say. Consider who you are *becoming*, focusing on your progress.

   Start replacing negative statements with positive ones, thinking about the kind of change you want to see in your life. You might reconceptualize your self-talk to sound more like "I am a work in progress, and that's totally fine." It's pointing you in the direction of achievable growth and is realistic. Another example is telling yourself something like, "Every moment I'm making an effort to be more conscious about how I manage my time." This statement acknowledges the fact that you are evolving and that you have a choice in creating a better future for yourself.

4. Putting feelings into words has tremendous therapeutic effects on your mind and brain.

FIVE

The Controlled
Emotions Mindset

Have you ever thrown a whole lot of clutter into a closet just before guests arrived—only to hear a loud noise as the closet door suddenly opened and everything fell out, in full view of your guests? The same thing can happen in your emotional life. If you repress and hide toxic emotions, the time will come when those buried emotions will suddenly come pouring out. And, of course, it will happen at the most inopportune time, because buried emotions are not controlled, thoughtful emotions. They are volcanic in nature and cannot be suppressed indefinitely. They will explode in some way at some time. They are also completely unique to you because emotions don't happen to you; emotions are made by you. You design the tectonic nature of your emotional experience.

When you express your emotions in a healthy way, you allow the free flow of neuropeptides and energy, which allows all bodily systems to function as a healthy whole. However, when you repress and deny your emotions, whatever they may be, you block the network of quantum and chemical pathways, stopping the flow of good chemicals that run your biology and behavior. You will be working against your customized, wired-for-love mode. When you do this for years, you are essentially becoming expert at not feeling what you feel, which in turn creates tremendous conflict in your mind and damage in your brain.[1]

Unfortunately, many of us have become experts at hiding our emotions—or think we have. Instead we create neurochemical chaos in our brains. Signs of suppressed feelings arising from this conflict include irritability, short temper, overreactivity, anxiety, frustration, fear, impulsiveness, a desire for control, perfectionism, and self-doubt.

Emotions are also fast. It takes about one hundred milliseconds for our nonconscious mind to react emotionally and about six hundred milliseconds for our conscious mind to register this reaction. By the time you decide that it's better not to get mad or be sad, your face has been expressing it for about five hundred milliseconds. But it's too late! The emotional signal has been sent. It's like pressing "send" on your text before you double-check the content and who you are sending it to. (See chapter 21 on memory for more on these numbers.)

We need to be very aware that the "repress" strategy should be used with caution because it doesn't do what we usually hope it will do—namely, make the pain go away, calm us down, reduce the aggression of a conversation, or stop a fight. Most of the time, we shut down out of shock, habit, or simply not knowing what else to do. However, it is actually a good idea to just say that you are angry, frustrated, sad, scared, surprised, excited, happy, calm, or whatever. Naming our emotions makes what we are thinking clearer to others—and to ourselves, because we often feel more grounded and more in control once we put words to emotions. This helps us to begin to process. And we give others the chance to respond and to empathize. This also stops us from assuming we know what others are thinking, because we don't. According to emotions expert Lisa Feldman Barrett, in her TED talk,

"Emotions are not what we think they are. They are not universally expressed and recognized. They are not hard-wired brain reactions that are uncontrollable."[2] She explains that we are not born with any prewired emotion circuits; we have the proclivity to the positive (I discussed this wired-for-love concept earlier), but through our choices (she calls these "guesses") we create our own emotions. What's more, her twenty-five years of research show that the billions of cells of your brain respond in the direction you send them: you are in control of building your emotions. This also means that your mind, not your brain, is in control, and that you are making predictions about your and others' emotional reactions with your mind, not your brain. Your brain is just responding. These predictions of others' emotions, and sometimes even your own, are not going to be 100 percent accurate. According to the laws of quantum physics, which work with predictions and probabilities, there is a 30 to 50 percent chance you will be wrong.

Acknowledging that you are expressing your uniquely created emotions in response to a particular situation is therefore an important step in detoxing your mind and brain. If you continue to try to hide what you feel, you will block your path to success in life.[3] If the acknowledgment of the emotions is leading to anxiety and accelerating the stress response, change your perception and build another replacement emotion by making it work for you instead of against you. Learn to make the negative energy into positive determined energy—reframe it. Through practice over cycles of twenty-one days (see chapters 20 and 22), you can learn new emotional patterns of responding.

We also need to stop thinking we can interpret someone else's emotions. That leads to a lot of problems and potential pain, because the emotions we seem to detect in others come from our own creative emotional perceptions. We can pick up if they are toxic or love-based, but we cannot pick up the exact detail. We simply cannot reduce emotions to a look in someone's face or body; that's only a part of the picture.

The knowledge that we have control over our emotions carries with it responsibility. It means you are responsible when you behave badly or explode emotionally. You are not at the mercy of preprogrammed emotion circuits that neurocentric approaches are dangerously trying to convince you of. This does not mean you deserve blame for your emotions; it means you need to take responsibility for how you are going to manage them so they don't carry into your future with negative effects. You are the only one who can change them. From my clinical experience, I found that once my patients grasped this concept, their progress was rapid. I have found that in my own life as well. This kind of emotional responsibility brings great freedom.

Controlled Emotions Mindset Activation Tips

1. The first vital step in controlling emotions is recognizing *you have control* over your emotions! You build them into your brain in a creative choice with your mind. They are not universal or preprogrammed; they are unique to you. Emotions don't happen to you; emotions are made by you.

2. The second vital step is to recognize you are not responsible for the cause of the emotion but rather for the management of the emotion.

3. It's important to protect your mind, brain, and body from keeping toxic emotions. Reframe toxic emotions and make them work for you.

4. Recognize the signs of repressed emotions and acknowledge them. This is the first step in detoxing your mind and brain of toxic emotions. (See my app on how to detox your thoughts at drleaf.com or your app store.)

5. You do not have to wear your heart on your sleeve or let everything hang out. But you do have to be honest with yourself.

Working out what you are feeling and how to deal with these emotions is an evolving process.

6. You need to express emotions appropriately, in an environment that is safe, accepting, and nonjudgmental. I suggest you create safe, less safe, and not safe people lists. The first group is people whom you know you can trust (loved ones, a really close friend, a counselor). The second group is people with whom you feel you can share to an extent, but not everything. The third group is people you definitely won't talk to because you know it will backfire.

7. Do not deny your feelings. Acknowledge them, face them, deal with them, and name them in a positive way as soon as possible—but most importantly, *when you are ready*. Remember, emotions are living and volcanic in nature and will explode somewhere sometime, very often when you least expect or want them to explode.

8. You are the only one who can identify your emotions, but the support from others can give you the courage to face and acknowledge what you feel.

9. Finally, don't think you know what someone else is feeling, because you will be 30 to 50 percent wrong and will cause increased emotional trauma to yourself by second-guessing in this way.

SIX

The Forgiveness Mindset

We're often told to "forgive and forget" the wrongs that we suffer, but it turns out that there is scientific truth (and gut logic) behind the common saying. Research shows that the details of a transgression are more susceptible to being forgotten when that transgression has been forgiven.[1]

Adopting a forgiveness mindset is a choice, an act of your free will. It comes with extreme health benefits. Forgiveness enables you to release toxic thoughts of anger, resentment, bitterness, shame, grief, regret, guilt, and hate. It disentangles you from the source of the issue, removing the negative energy from toxic thinking.

The emotions attached to the toxic thought can hold your mind in a nasty, vise-like grip. As long as these unhealthy toxic thoughts dominate your mind, you will not be able to reconceptualize your memories—that is, grow new, healthy thoughts.

Scientific research shows that forgiveness and love are good for your mind, brain, and body health! Ongoing results of the "Forgiveness Study" carried out by researchers at the University of Wisconsin found that people who develop an ability to forgive have greater control over their emotions; are significantly less angry, upset, and hurt; and are much healthier.[2] It's easier to move forward into a purposeful future when you have truly forgiven.

Forgiveness changes the brain. Research shows that forgiving someone increases the size of the brain's anterior superior temporal sulcus (aSTS).[3] In fact, the larger the amount of grey matter in this patch of cortex, the more likely we are to forgive those who have made a serious mistake by accident. The more you forgive, the more you are likely to forgive—the brain changes to accommodate a forgiveness mindset! This literally means the more you forgive, the easier it becomes.

Forgiveness is incredibly good for your health. Holding a grudge affects the cardiovascular and nervous systems, for example. In a study by the Mayo Clinic, people who focused on a personal grudge had elevated blood pressure and heart rates, as well as increased muscle tension and feelings of being less in control.[4] In this study, when asked to imagine forgiving the person who had hurt them, the participants said they felt more positive and relaxed, and had a greater sense of well-being. Other studies have shown that forgiveness has positive effects on our psychological health, which, in turn, impacts our physical health.[5]

But you may be thinking, *Caroline, you don't know what happened to me.* True, I do not, but I do know that holding on to your pain can negatively impact your health, blocking your ability to succeed in life. There's no single approach to learning how to forgive. As a human being who has experienced many painful situations, I know that grace and mercy do not always come easily. Yet it is not important how you forgive, just as long as you do—for your own sake as well as the sake of the people around you. Talking to a friend, therapist, or adviser (spiritual or otherwise) may be helpful during the process, allowing you to sort through your feelings.

Forgiveness does not make excuses for someone's behavior. By its nature, forgiveness acknowledges wrongdoing, *and*, at the same time, you choose to show grace and mercy. Indeed, forgiveness doesn't mean forgetting, condoning, or excusing whatever happened. Forgiveness acknowledges the pain and reconceptualizes it, releasing the heavy burden of bitterness and resentment.

Forgiveness Mindset Activation Tips

1. Forgiveness does not deny pain or wrongdoing; it is a *choice* to let go of the person who hurt you.
2. You can feel forgiveness in your body. Think of times in your life when you have forgiven someone and how it made you feel.
3. Forgiveness is not weakness but rather a sign of great courage and love. Think of how forgiveness can de-escalate negative thinking and negative situations. Think of this impact on those you are in relationship with.
4. Use all the mindsets discussed in this section to help you work on forgiving those who have hurt you.
5. Stop being angry and forgive, or you may become that anger— whatever you think about the most will grow.
6. Acknowledge the issue and the attached pain and anger you feel. You have to be honest with yourself if you truly want to forgive someone.
7. Recognize that healing requires time.
8. Reconceptualize the memory. Find a new way to think about the person(s) who hurt you. Think about the *context*. What was happening in that person's life when the hurt occurred? Why did they perhaps do what they did? What is their story? What is your story? Where are you in life?

SEVEN

The Happiness Mindset

Scrolling through Instagram, it is easy to believe that happiness means having a lot of money, nice things, status, or privilege. Yale's most popular class is on "happiness." Yet happiness is a much wider and more nuanced concept than our capitalistic society would have us believe. Happiness has more to do with a sense of inner satisfaction than external consumption. It is the joy you have living the "meaningful good life" and revolves around your ability to focus on the positive, to connect with others, and to have meaningful relationships in a community. Happiness is knowing where you belong and knowing why you are alive, regardless of your circumstances.

I cannot emphasize enough the importance of the link between happiness and community. Berkeley neuroscientist Emiliana Simon-Thomas has found that people with the strongest social connections are the happiest.[1] Our bodies respond positively when we become active members in a community. For example, the mesolimbic dopamine system, a system linked to addiction (which means to be consumed by something), lights up when we give to others, giving us a deep sense of pleasure.[2] We are essentially hardwired to love and serve others, which aligns with our wired-for-love design.

We also need to remember that happiness precedes success.[3] Working harder and achieving some entrepreneurial or academic or personal goal will not automatically make you happier. In a meta-analysis of 225 academic studies, researchers Sonja Lyubomirsky, Laura King, and Ed Diener found a strong causal relationship between happiness and satisfaction and successful business and life outcomes.[4] The satisfaction that comes from being truly happy plays a vital role in success.

In fact, every time you achieve success, your brain changes what success means to you, transforming with every experience, moment by moment, every day. You are constantly learning and growing. Happiness, satisfaction, and success are not static markers in a linear life; they are as dynamic and powerful as your thinking makes them. You are essentially in control of your happiness meter.

And happiness also does not mean a smooth and uncomplicated life, if such a life even exists. Harvard professor Shawn Achor indicates that increasing levels of happiness in the midst of a challenge, such as searching for a good investment in a down economy, results in success rates rising dramatically.[5] Challenges actually bring out the best in us. Getting to the other side of a challenge brings a sense of happiness in the achievement and sets the stage for the next challenge with the addition of the new skills you have gained from the challenge.[6]

The brain works significantly better when you *choose* to feel happy in the midst of a challenge. I have found repeatedly in my research and clinical experience and personal life that excitement rises when we adopt a positive attitude and persist in the face of a daunting task. Indeed, one of the greatest feelings in life is understanding something or completing an activity after a mental, and perhaps even physical, struggle. This leads to a sense of achievement as we rise to the challenge, contributing to our happiness. I always ask myself: *Do I want to give energy to the toxic situation by getting all worked up and not letting it go, or do I want to move all my mental energy onto a positive outcome that keeps my happiness meter up?* Your happiness level keeps you functional and moving forward.

We are not merely happy or unhappy. Our happiness does not depend on our circumstances. As Achor also notes, "It's a cultural myth that we cannot change our happiness."[7] A positive, love-based mindset and ability to make a stressful situation work for us is *completely* under our control and essentially how we change our happiness meter. Ultimately, as the poem at the beginning of this book declared, we are the "captain of [our] soul."

Happiness may seem to come easier to some people, but happiness is possible for all of us if we work on developing our wired-for-love, customized mindset (see section 2). Working on this mindset is less difficult than you may imagine. The simple act of writing down three things you are grateful for every day, for twenty-one days in a row, significantly increases optimism levels, and it holds for the next six months and even longer if you do this for sixty-three days (three cycles of twenty-one days)!

Laughter and play are wonderful ways to reduce toxic stress and increase happiness. Actually, all the mindsets in this section will increase your happiness meter. When we play, we stretch our emotional and expressive ranges. In fact, laughing is often referred to as "internal jogging" because it literally increases the flow of peptides and quantum energy in our brains and bodies.[8]

Many studies actually show why laughter deserves to be known as "the best medicine." It releases an instant flood of feel-good chemicals that boost the immune system.[9] Laughing also reduces levels of stress hormones. For example, a really good belly laugh can make cortisol drop by 39 percent and adrenalin by 70 percent and increase the "feel-good hormones," endorphins, by 29 percent. It can even make growth hormones skyrocket by 87 percent![10] Other research shows how laughter can boost your immune system by increasing levels of gamma interferon, which protects against respiratory tract infections.[11] Some studies even suggest that laughter helps to increase the flexibility of thought and is as effective as aerobic exercise in boosting health in body and mind. In fact, according to one study, laughing one hundred to two hundred times a day is equal to ten minutes of rowing or jogging! In sum, we shouldn't take life too seriously!

According to Robert Provine, "laughter is the archetypal human social signal and is all about relationships."[12] Provine's research found that people laugh thirty times more when they are around other people than when they are alone. This shows the entanglement we have in each other's lives.

Happiness Mindset Activation Tips

1. Choose to be happy, pushing through a challenge and enjoying the process of developing your understanding and abilities. If you fail, pick yourself up, even if you don't feel like it! Despite how you initially feel, choosing to be happy will become the energy source that keeps you going.

2. Think of having your own personal happiness meter—check it as often as you need to. If it's dropping then stop, breathe, and ask yourself why. Use the mindsets to help you work out the reason. Then choose to change it.

3. Be proactive in where you put your energy: you can choose to either bemoan and marinate in your misery or move your energy to do something constructive. It may be as simple as smiling at someone or taking your dog for a walk.

4. Don't allow yourself to think that *I will be so happy when this is over.* Enjoy the start, the middle, and the end! Tell yourself it's okay to experience different emotions, moving toward peaceful acceptance. You don't have to paint your face like a clown and pretend. You have to just be you, recognizing happiness is part of our wired-for-love design.

5. Choose to believe happiness is a possibility for you because you are wired for love. And remember, everyone has their own version of happiness and joy—one size does not fit all.

6. Make the effort to connect with others in a meaningful and deep way. Get involved in your community. Be social!

7. Watch funny videos, play a board game, watch a comedy, read a joke book, or make funny noises with your loved ones to develop and maintain a positive mindset.[13] Work fun into your daily routine and life. Having fun through play is the cheapest, easiest, and most effective way to increase happiness. It rejuvenates the mind, body, and the spirit and gets positive emotions flowing.

EIGHT

The Time Mindset

Our goal for positive changes and success should last a lifetime. We have to consider how we naturally think and how to use our thinking to achieve the lasting and meaningful success we are designed for. In today's instant culture, it's easy to forget this.

We all know that change takes time and that there are challenges on the road to success, but few are willing to persevere. Many of us do not fully understand the time it takes to change a behavior, which is why I emphasize the science of memory in this book (see chapter 21) and not just a neat, simple, quick-fix program that will guarantee instant victory. Success really does take hard work.

We have to remember that memories are thoughts. Everything we do is first a thought we build into our brains. The root of everything you say and do is based on the memories you have built into your brain through your thinking. Memories take time to build (twenty-one days to build a long-term memory and another forty-two days to build this memory into a thinking habit).

Nothing worthwhile happens in an instant. We can turn dreams into realities, but we first have to realize that it takes longer than the average one-second life span of a Twitter post to make a change. The technological age has brought with it a desire to see things, including change and success, as instantaneous. Yet there is no quick fix to success. Trying to make things happen fast and then giving up when they do not happen at the speed you have become accustomed to is unhealthy. It can cause you anguish and put your brain and body into toxic stress, keeping you stuck in a toxic cycle. But you can end this any time you choose.

Activating your brain through your choices allows it to build successful, meaningful memory. Like when you train your body to run a marathon or master a new exercise in the gym, your brain needs time to develop and achieve success, and you do this brain training with your mind—see this as mind cardio! We readily accept that it takes time to develop skill and expertise in a sport, yet when it comes to the mind, this wisdom often seems to disappear from our mental logic. Such a mindset leads to an endless cycle of cram learning for an exam or something needed for work and then forgetting most of it the next day.

Research on neuroplasticity, including mine, reveals that developing new habits takes cycles of sixty-three days at a minimum, not twenty-one days (see chapter 20). Most people give up within the first few days.[1] In my clinical practice I would start all my patients on one daily brief seven- to sixteen-minute mind detox exercise, partnered with at least one daily forty-five- to sixty-minute memory building exercise (they could do more if they desired). Within as little as three weeks, there was a transformation in their memories with observable change in their academic, work, social, emotional, cognitive, and intellectual performance. Real, long-term change that leads to transformed lives comes from persisting for at least three cycles of twenty-one days, so sixty-three days, since it takes about two months for new cells to form.[2] I saw this consistently over twenty-five years in clinical practice and research. There is no shortcut when it comes to mind and brain change.

Time Mindset Activation Tips

1. Don't let the time it takes for attaining a skill, changing a mindset, learning to control emotions, or forgiving discourage you from keeping on.

2. Don't sabotage yourself by fearing what other people will think of you or what other people will say about what you are doing as you go through the time-consuming process of change. Don't absorb toxic energy from other people.

3. Think of failure as knowledge obtained, even if it is knowledge of what not to do! Never label something a complete failure. Everything is a teaching moment developing your character.

4. New goals come with each new experience. It is good to have a goal and vision, but be prepared to adjust it, change it, or even do a 180-degree turn if necessary. Flexibility allows you to use your time effectively and enhances your progress toward success.

5. Understand the difference between distractions and being flexible. Flexibility moves you forward; distractions halt your progress.

6. Take the time to truly believe in yourself. If you don't have confidence in your abilities, no matter how skilled and talented you are, your performance will suffer. You may have to begin your journey to success with a sixty-three-day plan just to learn how to believe in yourself. You can find out more about this in my books *Switch On Your Brain* and *The Perfect You*.

7. Choose not to let time control you. You control time. Learn, as far as possible (we all have deadlines!), to flow with the natural sequence of time when you are completing a task.

8. Focus on the fact that it takes a minimum of sixty-three days to build lasting change in your brain. See chapters 20 and 22 for more details on this and apply it daily in your life.

9. If things take longer than you planned, adjust—don't panic. If you panic, you may end up undoing what you have just done!

NINE

The Possible Mindset

Do you see multiple possibilities in situations? Or do you see only what is in front of you as it is? If your plans do not work out, do you get thrown off? How? Can you shift from one possibility to the next?

Professor Achor shows that the brain's natural optimism bias is a great predictor of entrepreneurial success in school, work, and life. This optimism bias is the design of our brain that enables us to use our brains to perceive and pursue more than one possibility—we don't have to get stuck if things don't always go our way, because there are always other options.[1] We live in a world of probabilities, with the creative power in our minds to design blueprints of all these possibilities.

An entrepreneurial focus sees multiple possibilities in every situation; it is a mindset that perceives all kinds of probabilities and potentialities. This type of thinking is intrinsically hopeful; you just keep on trying till you find success. You appreciate the journey *and* the destination. And the good news is this is part of the wired-for-love nature of your brain and body—you just have to unlock it! Look at Thomas Edison, for instance. He tried about a thousand times before he succeeded in inventing the light bulb. When asked about his "failures," Edison declared that, "I have gotten lots of results! I know several thousand things that won't work!"[2] Edison didn't limit his potential to preconceived notions of success. He had a goal and he kept going until he achieved it, regardless of the number of trials along the way. He didn't see his attempts as failures; he saw his attempts as *results*. He had *gained worthwhile knowledge*—it was a learning process. Edison saw that what didn't work was as valuable as what did work. This is brilliant and this is key: attempts are not failures; attempts are results and worthwhile knowledge that has been gained. This is something I would work on a lot with my patients that made a profound difference to their progress.

When you *choose* to develop a mindset that allows you to perceive possibilities, the wired-for-love design of the brain is activated to respond, and attempts become possibilities rather than failures. This choice is a great predictor of success. I found this happening over and over with my patients and students in South Africa, where I worked for nearly thirty years. When they chose to adopt a possible mindset, they were able to persevere through desperate circumstances and achieve their goals. Their circumstances did not block their success; rather, where they were in life fueled their desire for change. They were learning how to learn, and nothing could stop them. Their determination impacted my own life and inspired me to continue teaching this message around the globe. Similarly, Achor, during his brief time in South Africa visiting some of the same schools, said he had never seen such determination and hunger to learn in a few sessions—the children he worked with in disadvantaged areas were more driven, disciplined, and grateful to learn than the privileged Harvard students he taught for a living (of whom one in four are depressed and not coping with their work-life balance)![3]

We cannot use our circumstances as an excuse not to succeed in life. It's not news to you that we all have issues we have to deal with and challenges we have to face. There is always something we are working on. Being able to see possibilities in the midst of your difficulties is, however, a game-changer. It transforms your thinking, allowing you to keep running your race. It is an essential mindset needed to succeed, even when you cannot see the end of the road—yet.

Possible Mindset Activation Tips

1. Tell yourself daily that attempts are not failures; attempts are results and worthwhile knowledge that has been gained.

2. Deliberately and intentionally practice seeing possibilities in every situation and write them down. The more you do this, the more you will find yourself applying these in your life.

3. *Choose* to develop a mindset that allows you to perceive possibilities, so that the wired-for-love design of your brain can be activated to respond.

4. Turn attempts into possibilities. Refuse to see them as failures. This choice is a great predictor of your success.

5. Stop yourself immediately if you catch yourself thinking and saying that there is no way out or that you are a failure. Replace with a statement such as, "I cannot be a failure because I am wired for success."

6. Make it a game to see how many possibilities you can think of for any one situation.

7. Train yourself to see a possibility as an opportunity, not a threat to shy away from.

8. Remember: we live in a world of probabilities and have the creative power in our mind to design blueprints of all these possibilities.

TEN

The Gratitude Mindset

I have been saying throughout the book thus far that we control our ability to thrive at school, work, and life, and gratitude plays a massive role in how successful we are. Of course, we all know how great we feel with an "attitude of gratitude." However, seeing scientific studies to support what we know instinctively is a helpful reminder, motivating us to change the way we think.

One recent study investigated the effects of gratitude on behavior and looked at the response in the brain to the mind.[1] The researchers found that subjects who participated in a gratitude letter-writing exercise showed both positive changes in their behavior and greater brain activity in the front of the brain (medial prefrontal cortex) up to three months later.[2] This study indicates that if we practice gratitude (remember the time mindset in chapter 8), we will revive the wired-for-love design of our brain, activating a self-perpetuating cycle of positivity in the mind.[3]

We should, of course, be highly cautious of reading too much into brain imaging studies—just because something lights up on a fancy machine does not mean that our brains are generating these responses to our environment.[4] It's our choices that determine

84

how we respond to the environment, and the brain reflects this in response: mind changes brain.

When we *choose* to be grateful, we tap into our natural design. Research on the effects gratitude has on our biology shows how being thankful increases our longevity, our ability to use our imagination, and our ability to problem-solve. It also improves our overall health.[5]

An attitude of gratitude leads to the feeling that life is worth living, which brings mental health benefits in a positive feedback loop that leads to more resilience, the ability to bounce back more quickly. I also found my patients with strong gratitude mindsets were more motivated to do the things that gave their lives meaning. This is in stark contrast to the negative feedback loop that a lack of gratitude sets up from becoming whiny; feeling "hard done by" or always the victim; always blaming someone, and becoming envious, jealous, and resentful of others' success. A study done in Japan found that those who experienced a life worth living— *Ikigai*—lived longer, healthier lives.[6]

Counting your blessings now makes it easier to recognize them later, because your mind will get better and better at the process of building a positive and grateful mindset. The more good you see in your life in the *now* moments, the happier and more successful you are likely to be in the future. As Willie Nelson once said, "When I started counting my blessings, my whole life turned around."[7]

Gratitude Mindset Activation Tips

1. Gratitude begins with an awareness of whether you have an attitude of gratitude, so intentionally and critically observe your thinking to determine if an attitude of gratitude is part of it.

2. Do you spend more time counting your blessings or more time focusing on what is missing from your life?

3. Are you thankful? Spend the next week analyzing how grateful you are. Keep a record, somehow, of every time you are grateful and every time you are whiny over a seven-day period. Tally it up at the end of the seven days—you may be shocked at the results!

4. Do you find yourself saying things like "We didn't manage to see that or do that" instead of "We did manage to see this and do that"?

5. Think about what you say before you say it, and if you have already begun to think something negative, watch what you say and catch those thoughts, change them, and say something positive before you start complaining and damaging your brain and your relationships!

ELEVEN

The Community Mindset

Human beings are social animals. Whether we like having alone time or not, we all need community. In fact, engaging positively with people in our social support network correlates with a number of desirable physical and mental outcomes. Community involvement has been associated with mental health and cognitive resilience, reduction of chronic pain, lower blood pressure, and improved cardiovascular health.[1]

Isolation, on the other hand, can negatively affect our well-being. Tragically, studies done on infants in custodial care indicate that a lack of human touch or contact can be fatal for newborns and young children.[2] Loneliness actually increases the risk for premature mortality among all ages, making it a growing public health hazard.[3] One recent study even indicates that social isolation and loneliness kill more people than obesity.[4] The researchers, looking at 148 separate studies representing some 300,000 participants, found that greater social connection meant a 50 percent reduction in the risk of an early death, while loneliness had the opposite effect. No wonder social isolation has been used as a type of punishment or torture![5] We should take the danger posed by isolation seriously—many nations around the world now suggest we are facing a "loneliness epidemic."[6] There is a desperate need for scientists to work together to make a community focus a public health priority.[7] This has become a quest in my work and something I speak about extensively: we are a team. To quote Mother Teresa: "I can do things you cannot, you can do things I cannot; together we can do great things."[8]

The more removed we become from human connection, the more potential there is for us to turn to the fantasy world as a replacement to reality, rather than using our imagination as a tool to create successful and satisfying lives. We all, to a certain extent, fantasize about how things could or should be, which often encourages us to pursue our dreams. Yet our imagination should not be divorced from real life, otherwise our fantasies can become more important to us than reality. This often leads to long-term social isolation that can dramatically affect our health and reduce our lifespan.

How do we combat this loneliness epidemic? Dr. Julianne Holt-Lunstad, lead researcher of the above-mentioned study on social isolation and longevity, argues that more money should be spent on shared social spaces such as recreation centers and community gardens, which are as integral to mental and physical well-being as eating a balanced diet and doing exercise.[9] She also notes that individuals should not only prepare for retirement in a financial way but in a social way as well—isolation can be particularly damaging to retirees.[10]

We can all actively pursue a community mindset. To this end, I also have a nonprofit organization called the Whole Mind Project, teaching "whole mind" and body health with a focus on community gardens, common meals, and love-based therapy, especially in churches, institutions, and disadvantaged areas.[11] Through these gardens and shared meals, and nonjudgmental shared listening, individuals learn not only how to eat in ways that nourish them and their community but also how to think in ways that change their lives and their worlds. We focus on spiritual, mental, and physical health being developed by the individual in community.

As part of our programs we have a Whole Mind bench, a place where individuals can come and talk about the issues they are facing in a loving, nonjudgmental, and peaceful environment. The Whole Mind bench is based on my research and clinical practice, as well as the friendship bench program that originated in Zimbabwe (a place where members of the community could come and discuss their problems).[12] It focuses on the context of an individual's problems and incorporates community-based healing techniques that focus on love and empathy.

Indeed, loneliness by its very nature is not something we can fix by ourselves. We have to reach all age groups and all spheres of society to combat social isolation and improve mental and physical health. As schools, universities, and workplaces are where individuals spend a meaningful portion of their lives, it is important to encourage social connectedness in these settings. We need to develop a holistic community mindset if we want to succeed in life and if we want to help others succeed in life as well.

Community Mindset Activation Tips

1. Think about what you could do to get out of the house and foster community in your area. Perhaps start a book club or arrange dinner parties and invite someone new each time. Get to know your neighbors and invite them for a walk or for coffee, or join a local community or spiritual center. The possibilities are endless!

2. You don't have to save the world; you need to start simply with purpose, and this can be as straightforward as looking outside your front door into your neighborhood, grocery store, gym, or church. If you are fulfilled on a personal level,

you will touch someone else, and this will spiral into a world effect. You matter, and what you think matters to your community and the greater purpose.

3. Join the Whole Mind Project: start a garden, build a bench, or have a dinner party! See our website for more ways you can get involved in what we do.

4. Volunteer! Serving others is a wonderful way to become part of a meaningful community, improving both your health and the health of your community.

TWELVE

The Support Mindset

An essential component to the community mindset discussed above is the power of healing in groups and reaching out to help others, as opposed to just getting help for oneself. High levels of social support predict longevity at least as reliably as healthy eating and regular exercise do, while low levels of social support are as damaging as high blood pressure.[1] For individuals facing difficulties in their lives (i.e., *everyone*), isolation can be lethal. Social support is crucial if we want to learn how to manage our emotions and deal with the vagaries of life.

Supportive relationships allow us to persevere through hard times.[2] One recent study found that social support was the greatest predictor of happiness during periods of high stress.[3] Stress can work for you or against you, based on your perception of the situation. Social support helps us deal with the challenges we face, because we realize that we do not face these challenges alone: we *see* our difficulties in a different light. In fact, in this study the correlation between positive social support and happiness was almost double the correlation between smoking and cancer.[4] This is an interesting comparison, because the causative link between smoking and cancer is largely unquestioned; however, the causative link between support and happiness is almost double but doesn't get as much attention! In fact, research shows that when we reach out to others in a supportive way, we increase our own healing by a factor of 63 percent.[5] We are designed to support each other!

Support is crucial in a learning environment. A 2011 study found that the more support a student *gave* versus *received*, the more positive his or her learning environment was.[6] Yet how often does a student help others when he or she is overwhelmed with work? In all likelihood not often enough, but those who do so are the happiest, which improves their academic performance. Likewise, people who pick up slack for others, invite coworkers to lunch, organize office activities, make sure that no one is left out, and are always willing to listen and help are ten times more likely to be engaged at work than people who keep to themselves, and are 40 percent more likely to get a promotion to boot.[7]

In my clinical practice, I always included a "help someone" aspect as part of any treatment. That is the principle of "get a session, give a session." Being supportive was an essential component in the patient's own healing and a means of increasing their intellectual performance. (This is part of the fifth integral step of the Switch On Your Brain 5-Step Learning Process you will learn about in chapter 20.) My husband, Mac, and I have brought up our four children to do the same. As a family, it is our second DNA to be helpers and organizers; we are always listening to and serving each other and the people we come into contact with. We always have a house full of people, and I wouldn't give that up for the world! We are a very happy family and obviously go through the "stuff" of life, but we deal with issues in a supportive and loving manner. But this didn't just *happen*. Mac and I chose to live our lives this way, and we work hard at this as a family daily. Based on both my professional and personal experience, I can say with certainty that applying the spiritual and scientific principle of helping others is incredibly powerful, therapeutic, and essential to thriving and succeeding.

Support Mindset Activation Tips

1. Look for every opportunity to support people in your circle of friends, acquaintances, and community.

2. When you feel burdened with work, emotionally challenged, or are going through something, try stopping for a moment and helping someone else, even if it is just to listen, hug, or encourage them. Send an email or text to someone, telling them you are thinking of them, or invite someone to dinner instead of eating alone.

3. When you are in a small space with a stranger, such as an elevator, smile and say hello instead of looking at the floor or your phone.

4. Choose to wake up every morning and ask yourself, *Who can I help today?*

5. Listen to others in a nonjudgmental, loving, and supportive way as often as you can. In fact, make this your modus operandi and watch your problems turn around. So: look at the person, and just *listen* and breathe until they finish, then ask, "How can I help you? What do you need?"

6. Always assume the best first. Create that positive energy, that "loveness." Don't jump to conclusions and assume the worst about a situation or person.

7. If you are not sure what another person thinks about you, or what the person meant by what they said, always assume the best. This will help you feel calm and steady.

8. Don't think you know what another person is thinking or that you can guess their emotions from their facial expressions. Always ask first. In this way, a person is made to feel

that they are important to you and that you care. We all need this, so give it 100 percent and watch it come back.

9. Everyone is busy, so we need to consciously make time for the people we love, because relationships take time and strategy, and you can't please everyone. So prioritize and strategize, but always be kind to everyone.

THIRTEEN

The Healthy Stress Mindset

I s the glass half full or half empty? Like everything in life, the way we view stressful situations can affect the way we deal with those situations. But stress is stress, right? Yes and no. Life can be incredibly stressful, yet the way you view stress can either make a difficult situation work for you or against you.[1]

If you face a difficult situation with a "glass half full" attitude, the blood vessels around your heart dilate. Increased blood flow results in increased oxygen flowing to your brain, which, in turn, increases your cognitive fluency and clarity of thought—that is, your ability to not only face a challenge but overcome it.[2] This increased blood flow also balances the sympathetic and parasympathetic nervous systems, allowing a number of neurophysiological and genetic processes to work for you, fueling intellectual growth.[3] A genetic switch will be turned on inside the hippocampus of your brain, which strengthens your body, allowing you to cope in a difficult situation.[4] Many neurophysiological responses will be activated, allowing you to stay strong amid adversity.[5] But if you see the glass as half empty, the opposite will happen, and stress will work against you.

I cannot stress the significance of perception enough. A 2013 study used two videos: one depicting stress as debilitating to performance and one detailing the ways in which stress enhances the human brain and body.[6] Participants who viewed the latter video scored higher on the Stress Mindset Scale—they saw stress as something that enhanced rather than diminished their performance, and their health and happiness improved. The intellectual performance and happiness of those who watched the video describing the debilitating effect of toxic stress, however, suffered. Worrying about stress will actually put your body into toxic stress, which will impact your mental and physical health. If you are constantly stressed about stress, stress will become an obstacle on your path to success. Changing your attitude toward stress is therefore essential to a healthy mental and physical self-care regimen.

But if stress can be good for us, why does it seem like everyone is freaking out about it? Why do they even sell adult coloring books for stress relief at the grocery store? On a daily basis, we are bombarded with news about the dangers of stress. When we read about the negative health effects of toxic stress, we certainly can get stressed-out about being stressed-out! It is like when we read about the dangers of not sleeping and how bad it is for us—and then we cannot sleep because we are worrying about not sleeping! Often there is so much emphasis on what is bad for us and what can go wrong that we forget to focus on what is good for us and what can go right.

But the good news is that you *can choose* how you view stress. You *can* learn to face a challenge and deal with it. You *can* learn how to not let stress defeat you! You can, as I love to say, freak out in the love zone!

Healthy Stress Mindset Activation Tips

1. See stress as something that enhances, rather than diminishes, your performance. Visualize those blood vessels around your heart dilating and pumping blood and oxygen into your

brain. Visualize neurotransmitters being released and see it all working together to help you focus and think with clarity to react in the best way.

2. See the situation you are facing as something you *can* handle versus something you can't handle; make stress work for you and not against you.

3. Each time you feel yourself teetering on the brink of toxic stress, speak with your friends or family (even if it is just a phone call!) to help you get perspective. And remind yourself that you can handle this.

4. Perhaps write down the benefits of a healthy reaction to stress and keep it on you, reading it when you feel challenged. Remember, you have an incredibly powerful mind!

5. When you face a challenge, tell yourself how good stress can be for you. Think of all the positive benefits (mentioned above) that good stress can have on your body. Tell yourself that you will have more clarity of thought if you make stress work for you.

FOURTEEN

The Expectancy Mindset

Expectations are part and parcel of everyday life. Consider the heightened awareness and excitement that comes from meeting a loved one at the airport over the holidays or receiving an anticipated birthday gift, party, or exam result. Imagine the intense satisfaction if the expectation is met or the intense disappointment if things do not go as hoped.

Due to the mind-body connection, expectancy produces real, neurophysiological outcomes in your body. Research indicates that *expecting* your physical work to bring about health benefits such as weight loss, for instance, brings about health benefits such as weight loss! In one study, eighty-four hotel attendants across seven hotels were split into two groups.[1] One group was told that the physical activity of cleaning their average of fifteen rooms a day, taking twenty to thirty minutes per room, met the Surgeon General's recommended amount of daily exercise. The others, as the control group, did not necessarily consider their work to be exercise. After four weeks the two groups were compared, and the results showed that those in the first group had lost

weight; their body fat percentages, waist-to-hip ratios, and sys-
tolic blood pressure had decreased. The hotel room attendants in
the control group, however, showed no improvement at all. These
changes occurred *despite* the fact that the hotel room attendants'
amount of work, amount of exercise outside of work, and diet
stayed exactly the same across both groups.[2] Expectations can
potentially affect the outcome of any given situation. If you are
expectant, you can change your brain and body in a positive way,
increasing the chance that what you hope will happen actually
happens.

How can you use your expectations to your advantage? Expecting that the effort you put into preparing for an exam, test,
or essay will pay off, or expecting you will have a good day, or
expecting things will work out in a relationship can change you
mentally and physically, *and* increase the likelihood of what you
hope coming about.

Think about the placebo effect, a well-documented phenom-
enon in which patients feel better after receiving a placebo, such
as drugs that are not really drugs but rather a harmless solution.[3] Jon Levine's study in 1978 regarding placebos was revolutionary at the time, because it suggested that patients don't
simply imagine or pretend their pain is eased with placebos.
His research showed that there is a measurable, physical change
with placebos, which is mediated by the release in the brain of
endogenous opioids called endorphins. Placebos can activate
endorphins, endocannabinoids (which bind to the same receptors as the psychoactive constituents of cannabis), or dopamine,
while reducing the levels of prostaglandins (which dilate blood
vessels and increase sensitivity to pain). Essentially, "placebos
can modulate the same biochemical pathways that are modu-
lated by drugs."[4]

Levine's findings have been corroborated by a number of
brain-imaging studies.[5] The mere thought that a treatment has
been received causes a beneficial physical response because of

the *expectation* that the treatment will work.[6] The individual's thoughts and feelings cause short-term physical changes in the brain or body because of the mind-body connection—even if he or she knows it is a placebo![7] For some people, even *knowingly* taking placebos may make them more aware of the role of the mind in, for example, controlling pain, and more inclined to believe that their thoughts could positively affect their mental and physical well-being.[8] What is fascinating in all these studies is that the inert substances are not creating biological changes; the active ingredient is a person's mind![9]

Placebos are made of words, rituals, symbols, and meanings, and all these elements are active in shaping the brain by creating expectancies.[10] The placebo effect is therefore an expectancy effect and has to do with the psychosocial context that characterizes the relationship between an inert substance and the patient and person in daily life.

The placebo effect can also, however, work in the opposite direction. In this case it is known as the nocebo (negative) effect.[11] While *placebo* means "I will please" in Latin, *nocebo* means "I will harm." Indeed, a person can experience harmful, unpleasant, or undesirable side effects after the administration of a placebo, *if* he or she believes that the fake treatment or drug will not work or will produce negative side effects. Bad expectations can create bad realities.

Our expectations change the structure of our brains. Therefore, learned associations result in real physiological and cognitive outcomes, such as more energy,[12] improved immune function, and improved mental and physical health, *if* these associations are positive. In essence, when we learn to expect good things, good things start to happen, such as better mental and physical performance. Yet the opposite is also true; thinking bad things are going to happen often allows bad things to happen! Fear is real and can build negative learned associations in the brain, which can affect our future thoughts, words, and actions.

Expectancy Mindset Activation Tips

1. Analyze your expectations. How have your expectations about a particular event or circumstance affected you?

2. Train yourself each day to go into superposition at least seven times a day and analyze whether you are creating a placebo or nocebo effect in your life. Do this for the small and the big things. Make it a habit.

3. Ask yourself: *Do I expect things to go well? Why? Do I expect things to go badly? Why?*

4. Take time to retrain your brain to an expectation mindset (see the time mindset above and chapters 20 and 22 for more on this).

5. Remember: the active ingredient of expectancy is your mind! This is so powerful, you will benefit enormously by just spending time on what this means for you in your life.

FIFTEEN

The Willpower Mindset

Are you one of those people who sets ten alarms at three-minute intervals just to get up in the morning? How much willpower does it take to get out of your warm, cozy bed? A lot, I know! Often, we have to push ourselves to do something we don't feel like doing. We all have willpower, because we all have things we must do that we don't want to do. Willpower is the mindset that allows us to persevere even if we do not feel like persevering.

If we harness our natural ability to persevere, developing our "iron will" like athletes before a competition, we can use our minds—that is, our ability to think, feel, and choose—to achieve our goals and be successful. If you *expect* that you will know the answers to a test because you have studied hard, for instance, you are more likely to study hard even if you don't feel like it, because your determination encourages you to keep on keeping on.[1] A willpower mindset is intimately connected to perseverance and is therefore directly linked to the expectancy mindset described above—it takes expectancy to the next level. Thinking you are limited in your knowledge is a limiting factor in itself, affecting your willpower and ability to concentrate and learn.[2] It is important to remember that your willpower is only limited *if you think it is limited.*

Willpower is especially important if we want to maintain a healthy lifestyle. There is the tendency to think that we will only lose or maintain our weight if we do physical exercise and eat less. Yet we will not develop healthy eating and exercise patterns if we do not have the willpower to keep exercising and eating right even when we don't feel like it. In reality, weight loss is more related to our minds and how much willpower we have than merely what we eat or whether we do yoga or CrossFit.[3]

We can use our willpower to change our *thoughts* about a physical or a mental act. These choices impact our brain and body, giving us the energy to pursue a task, achieve our goal, and succeed.

Willpower Mindset Activation Tips

1. Think of how you plug something into a wall to get it started. Now think of ways you can build up your willpower to do things you do not always feel like doing. What are your "plugs"? How can you motivate yourself to start, or finish, a task? Remember, this is a choice.

2. Observe your thinking and catch yourself when you feel like giving up. Think of how powerful your mind is and *choose* to persevere. Don't allow your feelings to control you!

3. Recall when you have expected and then used your willpower to push through. Relive this in detail. Analyze what you did and when, where, and how. Work out your expectancy-willpower pattern and watch your life change!

SIXTEEN

The Spiritual Mindset

For many people, spirituality is something that gives their lives purpose and shapes their thoughts, words, and actions. It colors their dreams and enables them to face whatever life throws their way. It can be a source of comfort during the hard times, peace when things do not go as planned, and motivation when they face a challenge.

In fact, spirituality can help us live long and successful lives. In the "blue zones," regions of the world with the highest concentrations of centenarians, spirituality is one of the key components associated with health and longevity.[1] It can foster a strong sense of community, helping people feel that they live for something greater than themselves and thus greater than their problems. Where there is purpose, there is hope.

Spirituality is not a "delusion."[2] Going to church, for example, can strengthen your immune system and decrease your blood pressure while providing a great source of mental and physical comfort.[3] Like everything in life, we can use spirituality in a negative sense, but the comfort and peace that comes with being part of a spiritual community can be invaluable.

I have found that science is not antagonistic to spirituality. For me personally, it is how I understand existence and the eternal nature of love, which I believe is God.[4] My spirituality is the guiding principle of my life. It gives me hope in a world that is often without hope and a sense of truth in relationship in a world where everything seems relative. It motivates my work, allowing me to succeed in life. I personally have found the meaning of love and God in science, and it has helped me see that love is the ultimate way to be truly human.

Spiritual Mindset Activation Tips

1. If you feel isolated and depressed, consider visiting a local place of worship or spiritual institution or group. If you look at local meetups, you may find at least one group of people whose spiritual philosophy may appeal to you. Explore!
2. If you are already part of a spiritual body or movement, try to participate in more community-based activities.
3. Read up on different religions and spiritualities and explore the philosophy behind their beliefs. Think of ways these beliefs can positively impact what people do and how content they are with their lives.
4. But most of all, choose to live in love. Choose to live a life of love that makes others feel loved. Your worldview or culture doesn't define you. It's love that does. Let's ask the question: What does love look like?

What's the Next Step?

The mindsets described above underscore the mind-brain/body connection. Mindsets are powerful and influential; they can be either energizing or draining; they can help or hinder you on the path to success.

Each of us has our own unique "flavor," our own unique way of thinking, feeling, and choosing, and this is reflected through our mindsets. Knowing about the mind-brain connection and the power of a mindset is central to understanding what successful living entails, but actually *applying* healthy mindsets in your life will only happen when you understand your identity. A powerful way to find your identity is through understanding your *customized* thinking pattern or your *customized mode of thinking*, which is the purpose of the next section.

This customized thinking, the way we each uniquely think, feel, and choose, characterizes our identity, and identity plays a major role in giving us a sense of purpose in life. This sense of purpose is critical if we want to succeed in life, because it helps us reflect on who we are in a deep and meaningful way. Finding identity is an ongoing but necessary process, and therefore has no time limit. It's essential we intentionally strive to understand and develop our identity for a multitude of reasons, because not only will it help us activate healthy mindsets and find purpose but it will also increase our health and longevity.[5] According to research, people who felt their lives had purpose and meaning reduced their risk of death by 15 percent.[6] Also according to this study, a positive mindset balances cortisol levels, which are important for healthy brain function and immune system regulation.

Viktor Frankl, a Jewish neurologist and psychiatrist who spent three years in a Nazi concentration camp, saw purpose and identity as life-saving. He later developed a form of psychotherapy based on his experiences.[7] The Nazis blatantly tried to dehumanize their victims by stripping their identity and therefore their meaning and purpose. Even the architecture at Auschwitz and Bergen-Belsen are shaped by a deep sense of purposelessness, meaninglessness, and hopelessness. Cold still pervades every corner of every room—I shiver when I think of the day I visited the camp in Poland. Yet, despite these terrible surroundings and despite the dehumanizing tactics of the Nazis, Frankl observed that some people were able to not only survive but hold on to their identity and sense of purpose in a collapsing world. Their sense of purpose helped them face, and survive, one of the worst atrocities in human history.

Purpose is incredibly powerful. In the late 1980s I began helping my patients understand their identity, their customized way of thinking, in order to give them purpose in a world that was making them feel like they did not measure up, that they were not good enough. Their inner conflict had dissolved into confusion, making them lose hope. Their loss of hope often developed into toxic mindsets, which often led to the very failures they believed that they were. When they began to realize that the way they thought was incredibly unique and powerful, they were motivated to change their mindsets to learn how to think and learn, and this was the point at which they began to see success in school, work, and life.

Motivated by the transformations I witnessed in my practice, I developed a series of Gift Profiles based on my research and theory that allow individuals to explore their customized, gifted mode of thinking. Once my patients (and now thousands of people globally who are also using my profiles) understood their customized thinking, it was so much easier for them to activate the power of right mindsets.

And now it's your turn to discover the wonderful way *you* think, your customized thinking, so that you can rediscover your purpose and release the power of your mindsets! In the following section, I have adapted one of the profiles I developed for my clinical practice—the Gift Profile—so that you can fill it in and interpret it yourself. This profile will help you understand the way you think, enabling you to apply the power of the mindsets discussed in section 1 to your life in *your unique way*. It will start empowering you to find meaning and purpose in your life.

SECTION TWO

The Gift Profile

SEVENTEEN

The Purpose of the Gift Profile

We each have an exclusive blueprint of thinking, a way of thinking that needs to be designed by us *for us*. It is called our "customized thinking" and is a gift because, the way we think is powerful and different from, but complementary, to everyone else's thinking—we are literally creating customized matter out of our minds. As we think, we create these customized exclusive realities. We need to understand and take advantage of our customized thinking in order to create meaningful realities filled with purpose. Understanding our customized way of thinking is in fact essential to understanding ourselves, our identities.

Thinking is a process and goes through a cycle, just like digestion. In the same way that food is digested and the nutritional content is used by our cells for life to take place, information has to be digested through thinking before it can be used in a "nutritionally" meaningful way, forming memory. Information that comes in through our senses is processed through our customized way of thinking. My customized thinking is different from yours—not better, just different and equally as wonderful. Completeness comes in these customized differences.

You will begin to discover your customized thinking when you fill in your Gift Profile. When you begin the journey of understanding and applying your customized way of thinking, you will think with more clarity and wisdom, activate healthy mindsets, build stronger memories, sharpen and develop your intelligence, improve your ability to communicate, and add purpose and meaning to your life.

In this chapter I will help you begin to understand your customized way of thinking. In the following chapter I will discuss the Gift Profile, and in the last chapter of this section you will improve your identity and self-esteem, see how this "nutritional content"—your customized thinking—can be used in a meaningful way in terms of activating mindsets and preparing for sustainable memory building. It is worth emphasizing that our ability to think, feel, and choose in our customized way is a true gift, enabling us to direct the course of our life with the power of purpose—the meaningful "good" life.

Customized Thinking and the Brain

Our customized way of thinking is the unique way each of our minds in action moves through the brain. Even though we all have the same parts and neurophysiology of the brain, there appears to be exclusivity in how and when different areas of the brain are activated, as well as diversity in the resultant growth of the dendrites on neurons in response to this activity (more on this in chapter 22). It's almost as though our brain tissue is arranged in a particular manner, matching our customized ability to process and digest information.[1] As the way in which we think, learn, and build memory enhances or damages the brain and body, it's wise to understand how our customized thinking operates and how to use it to activate the power contained within healthy mindsets.

We need to learn to capitalize on how our customized thinking works in our brains so that we can function at the highest level possible to achieve success in life. When we understand and learn how to make use of the unique customized way we think, we will feel at peace within ourselves as we draw on the power of healthy mindsets, becoming better communicators and improving our personal and professional relationships. We will experience a deep sense of clarity and discover our purpose; we will have a greater understanding of why we should get out of bed in the morning, doing daily activities that we find meaningful and engaging and that give us direction for our lives. Understanding our customized way of thinking is essential, not optional, for a life well lived. It activates the power of mindsets and drives the sustainability of memory.

No two individuals are alike. Studies of twins, for example, show us that even though they have identical DNA, they are different because they *think* differently.[2] Their customized mode of thinking, which results in a distinct way of building memory and therefore learning, changes their genetic expression, thereby changing what they say and do.[3] Twins, even if they are identical, can have incredibly different likes and dislikes, behavior, and life choices. They even have different susceptibilities to disease! Their differences can be studied by looking at their epigenetics, of which customized thinking is a part.[4] Epigenetics shows that externally driven changes, such as how we think and react to the events of life, will influence the behavior of our genes.[5] We are not merely our genes or our biology!

Customized Thinking and Genetic Expression

Changing the activity of the mind can alter the way basic genetic instructions are implemented.[6] The way you think is so powerful that it changes your genetic expression, constantly restructuring your brain.[7] It is exciting, empowering, and challenging to recognize that *you* are the one who has control over your thinking; you wield this power *through* the way you think, feel, and choose.

If you don't operate in your customized way of thinking, the bottom line is that you will work against who you are. Your mental and physical health will be compromised, because your thoughts can affect the way your genes are expressed. You can experience frustration, losing your clarity of thought and direction. You can lose your sense of inner peace, which in turn affects your sense of achievement. Your ability to communicate, learn, and function at school, at work, and in life can be negatively impacted.

Yet there is always hope. Fortunately, when you move back into your customized mode of thinking, you can literally repair your brain and body through your thoughts because of the neuroplastic nature of the brain.[8] Every cell in your body contains your full makeup of DNA.[9] Our thinking can actually switch genes on, influencing how the DNA functions.[10] The effective functioning of our genes is largely dependent on the effective functioning of our thinking, which kicks in when we learn how to use our customized way of thinking.

Instead of trying to think like Einstein, for example, we should recognize that Albert Einstein embraced his own unique way of thinking about and interacting with the world. His gift of thinking allowed him to develop his memory and release his genius, transforming the world of science. Who knows what you can achieve when you think and learn in your customized, excellent way—your gift? You would make a lousy Einstein, but you make a great you! You need to realize that you are wonderful just the way you are. We need to recognize the genius in ourselves as well as in each other.

Customized Thinking and Communication

In today's world, it often seems we do not know how to talk to each other. We all have different opinions; we all think differently; we all speak and act differently. Indeed, one of the greatest challenges can be interacting with people because they do not think like us! We can misunderstand what another person is trying to communicate to us, and vice versa. This misunderstanding often leads to arguments or worse.

When we understand how we think, however, we can recognize and appreciate that others think, feel, and choose differently as well. We recognize that these differences are not inherently bad but rather wonderfully good! We learn not to feel threatened by people who do not think, act, or speak like us. Turn this around and see it as enhancing your own genius—and this is exactly what research in mind and brain science is showing us. We will become more understanding, allowing us to develop and maintain a strong sense of community, which, as we saw in the mindsets section, is critical to human happiness and success. As social animals, we cannot function well if we cannot communicate.

Customized Thinking and Focus

When you learn how you uniquely think and learn—your customized thinking—you can maximize any situation by knowing how to get yourself to focus, pay attention, and concentrate on the task at hand. You will be able to make better decisions, learning how you function optimally in every situation. This ability to focus on a task and pay attention is an essential key to success in life, work, and school.

Indeed, understanding your customized mode of thinking, how you digest information, helps you understand how your mind works, thus activating correct mindsets. It allows you to utilize all your unique skills, talents, and abilities, which will not only lead you to success but help you define what success looks like in your own life.

Customized Thinking versus Neuroreductionism

The mind is separate from the brain. The mind works through the substrate of the brain, which, in turn, responds to the mind. There is a complex, integrated, and interdependent relationship between the brain and the mind that is not yet fully understood. The brain is like a complex quantum computer that reflects and expresses the mind or inner life of a human being. Every day we learn more and more about the nature of consciousness and how it affects cognitive functioning. It certainly is an exciting time in the world of science!

This way of thinking about the mind-brain relationship is, however, very different from the materialistic concept of the brain producing the mind (also known as physicalism).[11] In this latter view, the mind is merely the result of the firing of neurons; when these neurons eventually gain enough energy, they produce a conscious burst of mind as a side effect. This way of thinking about the mind-brain connection is known as *neuroreductionism*, because the brain is seen as the final answer to everything. Everything is reduced to the parts of the organ inside the human skull.

In this reductionistic worldview, we are just the firing of our neurons.[12] Free will and customized ways of thinking are irrelevant to the big picture, because we are confined and defined by our physical functions. Yet, as psychiatrist and mental health advocate Joanna Moncrieff notes,

> mental states are properties of living people within human forms of life expressed in activity that is purposive, interactive and whose meaning is inextricable from its social context. They are not abstract, context-independent entities like mathematical functions or chemical elements.[13]

We are not just biological automatons. We are complex, dynamic human beings that live in complex, dynamic societies. We shape our environments, and our environments shape us. We choose what to let into our heads; we choose who we want to be or become. We have a deep-seated sense of purpose that propels us forward, enabling us to change our society for the better.

So your amygdala *didn't* make you do it. Wait—do what? You are not your brain structures. Your amygdala, or any other part of your brain, for that matter, cannot make you say or do anything.

They do not control you; they are simply structures within the brain with specific neurophysiological functions that become more active *in response to* your expressing "what it feels like inside." They are activated by your unique perception, your customized mode of thinking.

Keys in the Dark

Imagine you are in a parking lot at night and you drop your keys.[14] You try looking for them, staying around the dim lamplight because that is the only area where you can actually see what is on the ground. Does looking under the lamplight mean that your keys couldn't be somewhere else in the dark? No, of course not. Similarly, our understanding of the brain is that limited. We often only look under the "lamplight," thinking that a brain scan can tell us all we need to know about being human, as though it can tell us where to find the "key." Yet we need to bear in mind that, notwithstanding the incredible recent advances in brain technology, quantum neurobiology, and neuroscientific research, scientists still do not fully understand how the brain functions, how it responds to the mind, and how we are all different, which is why consciousness is often referred to as the "hard question of science," a term coined by David Chalmers.[15]

We need to exercise caution when we read studies or articles on the brain. We should not get caught up in the excitement of striking fMRI images, hoping they will explain why we think what we think and do what we do.[16] In fact, a report from Johns Hopkins University showed that, of the more than forty thousand studies that have been published using fMRI technology, there is a 70 percent rate of false positives instead of the expected 5 percent.[17] A false positive may make it seem like an area is lighting up when in fact it's not, calling into question any conclusions made from that study.

Even the most detailed fMRI scan cannot show any more than the physical basis of perception.[18] We have to be extremely cautious in interpreting brain technology as a tool that describes the uniqueness of how we think. We are not the firing of neurons on a colorful scan. Brain technology merely demonstrates the global activity in the brain in response to when we think. In fact, an fMRI study on dead salmon was recently awarded the Ignoble prize.[19] Researchers showed pictures to dead fish, and this activity registered on an fMRI. In essence, it looked like the *dead* salmon was *thinking* about the pictures it had been shown! This study highlights the ridiculousness of a one-on-one matching of brain area and molecular processes to the unique and complex nature of human thinking.[20] If this kind of technology cannot always tell if something is alive or dead, we should not use it to make grand predictions about human behavior.

The Whole Brain and Thinking

What current neuroscientific research does indicate is that we can cause structural changes in our brains through the way we think, feel, and choose. Through our customized way of thinking, we can create matter with our minds.

When we think, all our cognitive abilities are involved, not just the areas that light up on a colorful scan. For instance, when we are introspective, employing what is called an *executive function*, the front part of the brain lights up more than other parts of the brain.[21] However, this does not mean that this is the only place where activity takes place when we perform this type of executive skill. The scan is not a uniquely exclusive window into what it feels like inside when we think deeply about something.

Brain technology records brain activity *in response to* the mind. It helps us learn about the brain, but it does not tell us about our inner person—who we are at our core. Our unique and wonderful way of thinking cannot be neatly packaged into separate parts that work independently of each other. Trying to pin down a specific area in the brain, with its molecular processes, to a thought or mindset is neuroreductionism at its peak, and falls within the realms of the neuromyths I spoke of earlier.

The Quantum Nature of Thought

As science progresses, researchers are getting glimpses into the minute, intricate structures of the brain that highlight the brain's complex quantum nature. This quantum nature responds to our customized mode of thinking, our innate, intangible humanness, which is impossible to capture on an fMRI. As Berkeley professor Henry Stapp, one of the leading quantum physicists of the twenty-first century, explains, we cannot use the same measures that we use to measure the physical world to measure the nonphysical world.[22]

Classical physics has no natural place for consciousness or the explanation of mind. It is based on a local and deterministic conception of nature that only works within the realm of the physical world, the 1 to 10 percent of what we can see.[23] But what about the nonphysical 90 to 99 percent part of who we are as humans?[24] What about the nonphysical world, which is the integral bigger part of our universe? When we talk about mind and consciousness, and when we talk about the brain and physical substance, we are addressing two completely different entities that require completely different conceptualizations and physics.[25] The mind requires a whole new way of doing science.

Sir Roger Penrose at Cambridge University, who is heralded as one of the greatest mathematicians of this century, argues that reality has a quantum character because thoughts share the same characteristics as quantum states.[26] Essentially, your customized thinking is your exclusive quantum state. Like a symphony orchestra, every structure in your brain has a unique role to play to make the music of your thoughts heard.[27] There is an infinite combination of possibilities that can produce a sound that is unique each time it is played *and* heard. In fact, the experience of the previous symphony colors the current symphony, providing a new level of complexity and quality. As the warm-up of an orchestra has no identifiable tune but is still an organized process, so is the warm-up cycle of our thinking: it eventually produces a product that is beautifully whole—a magnificent symphony and a magnificent thought.

Your customized mode of thinking can never be replicated or repeated because each experience you have had cannot be repeated. Indeed, reliving old memories or experiences adds a new layer of experience, rendering the old one as retold or reconceptualized. *Your* experience has already changed *your* thinking.

Essentially, every thought you have is a complex piece of music you have written with your choices, a piece that plays out in your brain and in your life. Mozart, describing how he created a musical composition, said that

> I keep expanding it, conceiving it more and more clearly until I have the entire composition finished in my head though it may be long. Then my mind seizes it as a glance of my eye, a beautiful picture, or a handsome youth. It does not come to me successively, with various parts worked out in detail, as they will later on, but in its entirety my imagination lets me hear it.[28]

Your imagination, as played out in your customized mode of thinking, allows you to hear, see, and experience *you*, just as Mozart's way of thinking allowed him to imagine and hear some of the greatest musical compositions in human history. No one can enter into your way of thinking and your experiences. Your imagination defies classical physics laws and explanations. It cannot be confined to the rules or bounds of the natural world that we can all experience, because it is your exclusive experience—it is *your* imagination.

Penrose uses Gödel's theorem, the incompleteness theory of the logician, to describe the quantum nature of thought.[29] In the simplest sense, this theorem shows that certain things, like understanding, are beyond the predictive power of equations. A computer, for instance, can be taught to play chess, but it does not understand the game. Understanding is a complex process that cannot be computed or mechanized; it is unique to each of us. After an appropriate amount of preparation, such as reading, thinking about, talking about, or listening to something, your unique perceptions express themselves through your thoughts, words, and actions, which are not measurable or restricted to an area in your brain that is common to all humans. As Dr. Seuss said, "Today you are You, that is truer than true. There is no one alive who is Youer than You."[30]

The Seven Modules of Thinking

The brain is a complex machine. In addition to the two hemispheres, four lobes, and numerous structures of the brain, there is an additional theorized arrangement of seven modules that run from top to bottom and left to right across the brain. It is theorized that our customized way of thinking is shaped by the way these seven modules of thinking interact.

Think of the seven modules of thinking as the components needed for a thought to be processed. Like our digestive process or the instruments of the orchestra in the previous example, all seven of these modules are activated in a way that is exclusive to us when we think. Our uniqueness is determined by how we *each* use *each* of these modules *and* by how they interact, which is different for each of us because we are different and have different perceptions and experiences.[31] Using the orchestra analogy, each violinist has a unique way he plays and interacts with his violin, as does every other musician.

We have to use all seven modules of thought to build a complete thought. We have to have all the musicians in the orchestra playing their part; we have to have all the parts of the digestive system at work. If we do not use them properly (which can happen with incorrect thinking), then we do not build the thought correctly. This may result in mental fogginess, lack of clarity, confusion, poor

121

memory, and even emotional strain—much like the cacophony that is the result of an orchestra playing out of sync; much like the pain we experience from undigested food.

Digesting Information

The way your brain responds to your thoughts has a specific structure, which can roughly be described as your seven modules of thinking working together in a customized way to build memories. To return to the analogy used at the beginning of this section, each thought is like a meal in your digestive system. In the same way that the several parts of the digestive system have specific roles and specific functions that allow you to digest a meal, so too does your thinking have specific parts and specific functions that allow you to digest a thought and build memory.

The seven modules of thinking are like the different parts of the digestive system, such as the mouth, tongue, stomach, pancreas, and colon. The mouth is the first part of the digestive system, the tongue and salivary glands are the next part of the digestive system, and so on. In a similar way, the seven modules of thinking are like the "structures" where different *stages* of thinking occur. Your thoughts develop as they pass through these seven modules. Just as food cannot be digested properly unless it goes through all stages of digestion, so thoughts need to pass through all the stages in order to be fully "processed." This process of digestion is unique to each of us, which is why I call this our *customized* mode of thinking.

The Science of the Seven Modules of Thinking

The seven modules of thought are based on research showing the general areas that the brain is divided into and how they respond to the mind-in-action.[32] The front of the brain responds to Intrapersonal type thinking and the back of the brain to Visual/Spatial type thinking, while other areas in the brain respond to

Interpersonal, Linguistic, Kinesthetic, Logical/Mathematical, and Musical type thinking.

In my work, I examine the relationship between the seven modules of thought and the law of diversity in the brain (see my theory in chapter 22).[33] No two people have the same thoughts about the same event or thing. Everyone's perceptions differ; each person has the power to create his or her own reality. In turn, the structural changes that occur in the brain in response to these unique perceptions will be different in each person. We each grow our own unique thoughts in our own unique way. This allows for an infinity of design within each of the seven different modules of thinking.[34]

The strongest evidence for diversity in the brain is our own instinctual awareness of self.[35] If you think of the million and one things that you know and think about and can do that no one else on the planet knows or thinks about or can do in exactly the same way as you, it is foolhardy to try to map how you think about *x* or *y* onto a specific area in the brain. If areas in the brain light up in a similar manner in someone who is completely different from you, what makes you different?

Measuring Your Customized Way of Thinking

There is no surefire way of measuring precisely how much of each of the seven modules of thinking you use as you digest information. Indeed, we do not know exactly how they work together; nevertheless, we are able to gain a certain level of insight into the way we think, and we can use this insight to our advantage. Even if we tried to use brain imaging techniques to decipher our perceptions, what we would see on these scans is the result of a general thinking pattern that brought a thought into conscious awareness in the first place. It does not show us the real-time, customized mode of thinking of an individual. Rather, these scans show the main focus of a task, such as reading or drawing, but not the thought process leading up to the task; thinking in real-time is extraordinarily fast (around 10^{27} operations per second) and virtually impossible to see with current brain technology. After all, the nature of thinking is infinite.

The Gift Profile I developed over twenty years ago and have expanded over the last ten years is a way of gaining insight into the mysterious world of thinking. Each module of thought is incredible, a veritable universe of constantly changing thoughts, and has characteristics that are distinctive to an individual, reflecting his or her moment-by-moment experiences. This is one of the many reasons that the descriptions and questions in my Gift Profile are broad and open-ended. You can use the profile to get a feel for your own customized mode of thinking, rather than discovering that you are "this kind of thinker" or "you do this because of that." Labels lock us in, causing the opposite of learning.

The scoring of the profile shows you the order of your thinking cycle (how you move through the metacognitive modules), which is your customized mode of thinking.

Each and every one of us thinks differently—but you don't need me to tell you that! The key is learning how to understand ourselves and deliberately apply this uniqueness to our everyday life, since these differences will affect the way in which we use our mindsets and learn and deal with what happens to us. We need to understand who we are, because we need to be *ourselves*, not someone else, to succeed in life. You will make a great you but a lousy someone else.

How the Seven Modules Work

The seven modules of thinking are Intrapersonal (introspection), Interpersonal (interaction), Linguistic (words), Logical/Mathematical (rationalization), Kinesthetic (senses), Musical (intuition), and Visual/Spatial (imagination).[36] It is theorized that brain tissue is clustered into these seven modules, which stretch from top to bottom and left to right across the brain. They are not fixed sections; the metacognitive modules flow into each other, working together, especially when the brain has been damaged.

Each metacognitive module has a general umbrella-type function. The front of the brain becomes more active with introspection, decision making, planning, deep analysis, shifting between thoughts, forming goals and sticking to them, developing strategies, and so on. This is called the *Intrapersonal* module of thinking. Just behind this area is the *Interpersonal* module of thinking, which becomes more active in response to social interaction, communication, turn-taking, and tuning in to the needs of others. This is followed by the *Linguistic* module of thinking, which becomes more active with spoken and written language. Then comes the *Logical/Mathematical* module of thinking, which becomes more active with reasoning, logic, scientific type thought, numbers, and problem solving. Next is the *Kinesthetic* module of thinking, which is more active with physical activity and body awareness. The *Musical* module involves instinct, musical talent, and reading between the lines. Finally, there is the *Visual/Spatial* module of thinking at the back of the brain, which is more active when we imagine and form mental maps in our mind.

As you process information, quantum action occurs, activating a unique response that is reflected in how you use your seven modules of thinking. What is the result? You use all seven types of thought in your own customized way, like a filter or a well-worn pathway. It feels "natural" to think in this way.

As you think in your own customized way, your brain kicks into high gear and you operate like a fine-tuned car with all seven types of thought oiled into thinking "it" through. When this happens, all kinds of wonderful chemicals flow through your brain, and a frenzy of high-level thinking and memory building begins!

My theory, the Geodesic Information Processing Theory (see chapter 22) looks at the neurological impact of this process of thinking—that is, the mind-brain/body connection. It takes into consideration the fact that the brain can change (neuroplasticity).

Instead of describing a person according to a particular facet, such as linguistic or auditory, the Geodesic Information Processing Theory behind the Gift Profile describes an individual in terms of his or her combination of the seven different modules of thinking— the whole being made up of the parts.

Customized Thinking in the Corporate World, an Example

I am often asked to help business leaders develop their thinking and learning skills. One of the most interesting experiences I have had was in the middle of a problem-solving activity at a company. It became very obvious that some of the individuals I was working with had little understanding or grace for each other's differences. This particular company was also going through a period of great stress, and it also became obvious that some of the problems it was facing as a business could be traced to the problems the employees were having with one another.

On one side of a huge conference table sat a guy who was about six-foot-eight and looked like he could play professional football. He had an obvious dislike for a colleague who was sitting directly across the table from him and who was around five-foot-two. There was a definite physical disadvantage between the two men. As we were working through several problem-solving exercises, the tension between the two men just kept increasing and increasing. Finally, the taller of the pair leaned across the table, enraged by something the shorter man had said. I realized that in order to avert a brawl it might be wise to use that moment as an illustration of how important it is to understand that even though we are each wired differently, we are all wired for success.

I asked both men to look at their Gift Profiles to see their different ways of thinking and Gift Profile learning. It turns out (perhaps not surprisingly) that they were polar opposites. The one man would focus and pay attention with movement and imagination, communicating through action what he saw in his mind's eye.

His counterpart, on the other hand, used reasoning and words. The smaller gentleman was always trying to speak persuasively, but he was just speaking the big gentleman across the table into an absolute frenzy. Once I had shown them the differences in the structure of their learning patterns and how to better understand each other, the light bulbs switched on, and by the end of the training session they walked out arm-in-arm, talking about an issue in their department!

Getting these two gentlemen to understand how they each thought and learned differently helped them realize that they were not a threat to each other, which was key in changing the relationship. They were radically able to improve the way they communicated with each other, even gleaning valuable wisdom from what the other had to say.

Research shows that when we think properly—that is, when we think in our customized mode—we are better at analyzing a difficult situation. We are able to generate new knowledge and categorize facts in a speedy manner, not allowing our emotions to get the better of us. If we could all apply this in our lives, imagine the kind of world we would live in!

EIGHTEEN

The Gift Profile

N ow you are ready to dive into your own Gift Profile!
To get the most out of this Gift Profile, you need to really
think about your thinking, which is why the first section of this
book is on *mindsets*.

It is also incredibly important to remember that none of the
seven modules of thinking operate in isolation; indeed, their power
comes from their interaction. As the saying goes, the whole is
greater than the sum of the parts. The challenge is how to discover
what your combination is, your "story of the sum," in the Gift
Profile. For an in-depth exploration of your identity using the seven
modules of thinking, you can look at my book *The Perfect You*,
which includes the Unique Qualitative (UQ) Assessment Tool,
another questionnaire that will teach you how to self-reflect in
a quantitative, open-ended way. It will also help you understand
your unique identity as a blueprint that develops over time. In this
book, however, I use these seven modules of thinking in a different
way to help you explore and understand your customized thinking
using the Gift Profile.

When it comes to filling in any type of profile, we always need to bear in mind that there is no single profile assessment or test that can define the complexity of humanity. The slice of information measured in any form of assessment is so very thin compared to the entirety and complexity of who each one of us truly is. The IQ movement has misled us to believe that we are either gifted or not gifted, that we either have a high IQ or a low IQ, that we either can or can't go to college, that we are either below average, average, or brilliant. Indeed, many people have been incorrectly led to believe that intelligence is determined between ages five and seven and nothing can change this. Fortunately, this bleak outlook is incorrect.

We are often erroneously grouped into boxes such as learning disabled, ADHD, gifted, right-brained, left-brained, overachiever, underachiever, intelligent, or low-functioning, and these definitions can quickly become a part of how we see ourselves—our sense of self-worth. Labels can easily wall us in and restrict us. Yet our customized way of thinking is so much more than what any label can say about us. We are not a number or a category; we have no competition.

Thankfully, the world of science is changing. Research shows that intelligence is unique to each of us. Talent is not fixed; it grows and develops with us as we use it. You are as intelligent as you want to be! You have had this natural power inside you all along; you just have to learn how to use it. Wherever you are in in your life, you can grow and develop into who you were designed to be.

How to Use and Interpret the Gift Profile

The three tables below will help you understand and use the Gift Profile. The first table contains the definitions of the seven modules of thought. Following this table is an image that will help you visualize the modules in the brain. The second table describes the seven stages of how a thought is digested—that is, the cycle of thinking. The third table describes the scoring method for the profile. There is also an *explanation* of how to fill in and interpret the profile below the tables. These tables are followed by the actual Gift Profile.

Table I: The Seven Modules of Thinking

Module of Thinking	Description
Intrapersonal (Introspection)	Deep thinking, analyzing, thinking things through in your head
Interpersonal (Interaction)	Communication, conversations, and sharing information
Linguistic (Words)	Spoken and written words
Logical/Mathematical (Rationalization)	Scientific and strategic reasoning, order, and planning
Kinesthetic (Senses)	Movement, experiential, and body-awareness
Musical (Intuition)	Instinct, reading between the lines, and musical talent
Visual/Spatial (Imagination)	Imagination, or seeing "in the mind's eye"

Image 18.1

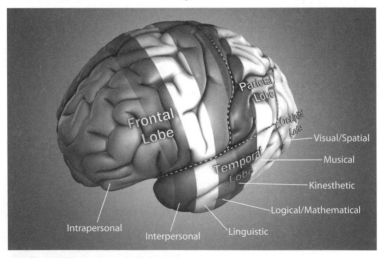

The seven different types of thinking

The Cycle of Thinking

As explained in the preceding sections, each one of us has seven stages that our thoughts sequence through in order to digest information. This sequence is called the *cycle of thinking*. Our uniqueness comes in which module of thought we use for which stage of the cycle. The process is different for each of us. For example, one person may use Intrapersonal for stage one, and another person may use Kinesthetic for stage one. However, until we move through *all* of these seven stages—each in our own way—the thought will not be fully processed. In other words, we won't be thinking properly unless we move through all seven stages of the thinking cycle.

Obviously, this process is incredibly fast, so you will not *feel* it happen. According to anesthetist and researcher Dr. Stuart Hameroff, we have conscious bursts of activity around forty times a second.[1] We experience these bursts like a cartoon strip where all the individual frames are experienced as a conscious event about every ten seconds, somewhat similar to watching a cartoon movie. We have an estimated six of these conscious bursts in a minute, around 360 per hour (6 × 60), and 8,640 every twenty-four hours (360 × 24). On the nonconscious level of mind, intelligent thinking occurs at about a million operations per second (and general activity occurs at about 10^{27} operations per second).[2]

Memories with sufficient energy move into the conscious mind at a rate of about five to seven in approximately five to ten seconds, sometimes quicker, which equals around eight thousand thoughts every twenty-four hours.[3] These thoughts are triggered by internal memories and external stimulation from the environment; they are part of your perception and provide context.

Totaled together, we have anything from an estimated sixteen to eighteen *thousand* thoughts moving through our head every day! These thoughts include processing (building new information into memory) thoughts and contextual (informational) thoughts. According to the National Science Foundation, we think fifty thousand thoughts per day.[4] This may be possible, especially in light of what we know about the power of the nonconscious mind, yet a lot more research needs to be done in this area.[5]

There is no need to be concerned, therefore, if you do not feel a thought going through the seven modules. In fact, if you do feel it, you may want to be concerned because your thinking is too slow! We also cannot remember everything and we are not supposed to; we remember what we pay attention to and what we feel we need to remember in the moment.

Even though it interesting to conjecture about numbers, which underscore how important it is to control what we let into our heads, we should not get too hung up on or concerned about them. Instead, we should focus on the enormity of the power in our non-conscious mind and learn how to use that power more effectively.[6]

It is important to remember that although our thought-life is a "stream of consciousness," with thousands of individual thoughts blending together, we can control what we allow into our heads. We are able to evaluate the individual frames of thought by self-regulating our stream of consciousness. When we get distracted by external influences and toxic reactions to life, however, our ability to self-regulate can be affected, with negative consequences for our mental and physical health. By training ourselves to understand our customized way of thinking, we are *retraining* our self-regulatory function, which allows us to monitor and observe our thinking.

In terms of the cycle of thought, you will only really be aware of your first two types of thought among the seven modules, and perhaps your last two in your order. The process is just too fast and there is just too much going on for you to be cognizant of every-thing. This is often why people describe themselves as "visual" or "auditory" learners, because that is what they are *aware of*—but this is not what is really happening. This narrow way of approaching learning is known as *learning styles theory*. These kinds of state-ments and beliefs are incorrect and reductionistic; it is impossible to just use one module of thought as you learn and build memory.

According to learning styles theory, if a student self-identifies as a visual learner, content should be presented to them visually and not auditorily. However, the differences we see among ourselves are never as black-and-white as "this person is a visual learner" and "this person is an auditory learner."

A recent meta-analysis evaluated findings from a number of studies testing learning styles theories.[7] The researchers concluded that there was an insufficient evidence base to support learning styles application to educational contexts. The common VAK (Visual, Auditory, Kinesthetic) learning styles theory, for instance, suggests that each student has one favored modality of learning and that teachers should identify students' preferred learning styles and create lesson plans aimed at these learning styles. Yet this is almost impossible to implement considering the size of classes and the demands of an educational day, and it has been shown to have minimal value in terms of memory formation.[8] Additionally, there is a sore lack of empirical evidence for assessing these so-called learning style preferences. Because of this lack, using learning styles to inform instruction in order to improve student outcomes at school and university raises concerns about the pervasiveness of the theory. Its near universal impact on current classroom and corporate environments is a problem.[9] The limited time and resources available in the world of education should be aimed at developing and implementing truly evidence-based interventions and approaches.[10]

I have trained thousands of teachers in my career in the United States, South Africa, and other parts of the African continent. One of my overriding objectives has been to dispel this learning style neuromyth and set learners free. We should not approach learning with the preconception that there is "thinking inside the box" learning and "thinking outside the box" learning. As the "gangsta gardener" Ron Finley says, when it comes to the human imagination there isn't a box to begin with.[11] Your mind is incredibly powerful and complex; you are not just one thing. Your powerful and complex thoughts are a combination of at least seven processes that you use in your own unique way. Your cognitive strength lies in the sum of *all* your parts—and no one on this planet thinks like you do.

Table II: The Cycle of Thinking

Steps	Description	Feels Like
1. Focus Become consciously aware of taking in information.	Information comes in through your five senses and activates existing thoughts in your mind.	This is experienced as an awareness of gathering information and the activation of thoughts in your mind just on the tip of consciousness. It is literally the doorway allowing information into your mind.
2. Attention Become consciously aware of being absorbed by the information.	You build connections to this information from existing information and memories. These connections help your mind make sense of new information. You start to build a temporary memory.	This feels like a deliberate and intentional choice to set your mind on the incoming information.
3/4/5. Analysis Consolidate/confirm/integrate on a nonconscious level—not fully aware.	You consolidate this information in the "trees" (neural networks) in the cortex of your brain. You confirm this information and decide if you feel it is true and/or accurate. You integrate the information into the networks of your memories.	You may or may not experience this as a quick burst of thinking, feeling, and choosing because it's so quick.
6. Apply Become consciously aware of the new information.	The incoming and upcoming information takes on meaning.	You experience this as a feeling of "This is meaningful; I can use this or do this."
7. Close Become consciously aware of the need to do something.	You get a sense of closure leading to some sort of action that restarts the cycle.	You experience this as some sort of action.

There is an actual order, a beautiful structure, to how you use the modules to think in your customized way. Your brain is designed to reflect this way of thinking and learning, which is what you will begin to discover in the Gift Profile. As you become aware of this order, using your customized mode of thinking, you will start recognizing how you "think through" information, which will help you intentionally use and develop your thinking pattern at school, at work, and in life.

How to Fill In the Gift Profile

If you are feeling a little confused at this point, no problem! As you fill in the Gift Profile, things will begin to fall into place. I am just giving you information at this point to prepare you for the profile, which is coming up in the next section. I encourage you to flip back and forth, rereading these descriptive sections and the earlier sections of the book along with the Gift Profile to help you understand this magnificent truth: you have a unique, customized way of thinking.

I have created a simple profile with seventy questions, which I call my abridged Gift Profile. The fuller Gift Profile is beyond the scope of this book but can be found on my online app, Perfectly You.[12] Both are adapted from the original profile (over one thousand questions!), which I developed and used in my clinical practice for twenty-five years. I love this Gift Profile for many reasons, not least of which is that it has helped so many people realize the power and uniqueness of their minds, but the fun part is that there are *no wrong answers*. You either answer yes or no—both are correct because this is not a test of your knowledge base. The profile is an exploration of how you think, feel, choose, and learn—your customized thinking. Whatever scores you get are *all* good because they simply reflect the *order* of your thinking cycle and not your skill level. So, 30 percent is as good as 100 percent—it just shows the order you move through the brain.

Remember, you use *all* of the seven types of thinking in your customized thinking. Your highest score is the type of thought you will draw on first; it is literally the doorway to how you get information into your mind. The second highest score is the thinking you draw on as you intentionally choose to set your mind on the incoming information. The third, fourth, and fifth scores draw on the types of thinking that will start the analysis part of thought digestion, and is so quick you may or may not experience it as a rapid burst of thinking, feeling, and choosing. The sixth score is how you apply the new information. You experience this as a feeling of something like "This is meaningful; I can use this or do this." Finally, the seventh score shows you how you bring closure to a cycle of thought as understanding begins to form; you may experience this as some sort of action.

It's really important to understand that your highest score *does not* describe the entirety of who you are. All seven scores are the ingredients of how you think and how your brain responds to how you think. You have to use all seven modules to think, and the more efficiently you use them, the better you will function in school, work, and life. The Switch On Your Brain 5-Step Learning Process, which you will learn about in chapter 20, activates your customized thinking to produce the strongest memories and is therefore very complementary to the development of your mind.

Filling In the Abridged Gift Profile

Below are several tips to remember as you fill in your Gift Profile.

- The Gift Profile in this section is the abridged version of one of my original profiles. It is the shortened version and is therefore just an indication or a sampling of your thinking cycle—it is not comprehensive. (For the more comprehensive profile, see the Perfectly You online program, www.perfectlyyou.com.)

- It is in a questionnaire format, arranged in seven different categories, each of which represents one of the seven modules that make up your customized way of thinking.
- There is *no* wrong answer. All answers are correct.
- The more quickly you answer the profile, the more accurate the answer. If you find yourself debating whether this is like you or not, then it's most likely not and you should circle no.
- You are not trying to impress anyone—pure honesty is what is required.
- You are not supposed to score high on everything; you are using the scores to look for your thinking order—not your skill level—so any score you get is brilliant because it describes you!
- The highest score is the entry point of information, how you gather information; the middle five scores are how you build short term memory and analyze; the last score is how you close the cycle. Then the process starts all over again, and again—all day long, as you build knowledge into your brain in your customized way.
- The scores will range from high to low, showing where your thinking cycle starts and ends; they reflect your order and which pillar in the brain is being activated in response.
- Because there are differences even within the similarities, two people can have similar strengths, but by asking yourself more specific questions, the differences within your similarities will become obvious.
- When answering the questions, simply select a yes or no answer to each question. Circle yes if you think the question applies to you. Circle no if it does not. Some questions may seem ambiguous, in which case you should follow your gut instinct, circling yes or no according to your initial reaction.

- When finished, simply add up your circles per section (there are seven sections, one for each type of thinking) and convert to a percentage (e.g., 7/10 = 70 percent).

- Line up the scores from highest to lowest to find your customized mode of thinking.

- If you feel that you think differently in different areas of your life (such as when you are at home compared to when you are at the office or school), you have detected something very interesting at the heart of your customized thinking. Each of us has a true self, and each of us also has an adapted self that has been influenced by our environment and circumstances. We have learned different skills; we are designed to adapt our gifting to our particular environment. Therefore, you may wish to complete the Gift Profile twice, once from a personal point of view and once from a professional and/or academic perspective. For example, as you are completing the Gift Profile, you might find yourself thinking, *I don't really like doing this, but I have had to learn the skill,* or *This doesn't come naturally to me, but I have developed this skill over the years.* The most accurate profile will be the personal one. Most of the time they will be almost identical. If they are very different, you may be following the wrong path—a bit like trying to fit a square peg in a round hole—something to ponder.

- If you get the same score on two or more of the modules of thinking, then all you need to do is go back over the questions a second time in a very deliberate and intentional way, asking yourself something like *Is this who I really am, or is this what I have had to learn to do/think because of my environment or circumstances?* In this way, you will tease out the real you, which should alter the scores. You may have to do this a couple of times because sometimes we have habituated behavior because we needed to adapt, but it does not feel like the real you.

- As you complete the profile, try to stand outside yourself and observe your own thinking. You are actually designed to do this! The frontal lobe responds and fires up when you think about your thinking. I call this the MPA (multiple perspective advantage—see chapter 3). Use these questions to guide you as you use your MPA:
  - What do I like to do? (If you don't like it, don't select it!)
  - What comes naturally to me?
  - What appeals to me?
  - What feels comfortable and normal?
  - What feels like me when I am thinking things through?
- The second time you complete the profile, keep the following questions in mind:
  - What have I had to develop to perform better at school, work, or life? (For example, you may not naturally be rigidly organized but you have had to train yourself in order to cope with your job.)
  - How has a particular skill or quality developed due to the nature of my work, school, and life demands?
  - What is it that I don't like to do but have had to do or have learned to do in my work, school, or living environment?

In summary:

- There is no right or wrong answer.
- You are not trying to impress anyone.
- Pure honesty is what is required.
- You are not supposed to score high on everything—it's not a test and you are not being graded! You are simply looking for how you move through the cycle of thought.

Most of your modules of thinking will probably score around 40 to 70 percent; a few will be around 70 to 80 percent and two or three may be higher. Some modules may even be as low as 15 to 20 percent—this not a problem, weakness, or failing! Remember, the Gift Profile simply tells you the order you move through your thinking cycle. There are no right or wrong answers. The lowest score tells you how you close your cycle of thought, launching you into the next cycle; the highest score tells you how you focus, and so on (see Table II above). If you get a high score in most areas, you have either mixed your personal and academic profiles or you have not been totally honest! If this happens, redo the profile, taking time to deliberately answer the questions.

Once you have filled in and scored your profile, come back and fill in the chart below (Table III).

Table III: The Sequence of Your Thought Cycle

Order/Sequence	Percentage	Thinking Module
First highest		
Second highest		
Third highest		
Fourth highest		
Fifth highest		
Sixth highest		
Seventh highest		

Now you can finally complete the abridged version of the Gift Profile!

The Gift Profile

1. Intrapersonal/Introspection Module of Thinking

1. Do you find it easy to stand outside yourself and observe your range of emotions? YES/NO

2. Do you find you need multiple ways of expressing your emotions? YES/NO

3. Do you find your internal life fascinating? YES/NO

4. Do you find yourself focusing in on your internal thoughts quite frequently—switching off to the external and switching on to the internal? YES/NO

5. Do you work well on your own? YES/NO

6. Do you find yourself pondering the deep questions? YES/NO

7. Do you like to spend time in your head? YES/NO

8. Do you find it easy to spend time alone? YES/NO

9. Do you find it necessary to look away as you process information? YES/NO

10. Are you determined to make a difference in life? YES/NO

Score:	*Example:*
1. Count the number of yesses	1. 7 yesses
2. Multiply by 10	2. 7 × 10 – 70
3. Add percent sign	3. 70%

2. Interpersonal/Interaction Module of Thinking

1. Do you feel tuned in to others? YES/NO

2. Are you sensitive to others' emotions and moods to the point where you pick up on them, almost exhausting yourself feeling them? YES/NO

3. Do you find yourself watching people and their reactions? YES/NO

4. Can you put yourself in other people's shoes? YES/NO

5. Can you motivate others? YES/NO

6. Are you good at networking with and between others? YES/NO

7. Do you like people around you a lot? YES/NO

8. Do you like to negotiate? YES/NO

9. Are you a peacemaker? YES/NO

10. Do you notice if others don't understand you and can you revise what you are saying and/or explaining if you notice they don't understand you? YES/NO

Score:

1. Count the number of yesses

2. Multiply by 10

3. Add percent sign

3. Linguistic/Word Thinking Module

1. Do you love playing with words? YES/NO

2. Do you prefer emailing or texting to talking on the phone most of the time? YES/NO

3. Would you consider yourself skilled at using language to communicate? YES/NO

4. Do you feel you need to use lots of words to communicate? YES/NO

5. Do you need to express yourself or explain yourself through speaking and writing lots of words? YES/NO

6. Do you read a lot? YES/NO

7. Do you like telling stories? YES/NO

8. Do you consider yourself to have good general knowledge? YES/NO

9. Do you seem longwinded to people when you explain things? YES/NO

10. Do you feel you need to provide a lot of context with words when you talk? YES/NO

Score:

1. Count the number of yesses
2. Multiply by 10
3. Add percent sign

4. Logical/Mathematical/Rational Module of Thinking

1. Do you naturally find yourself reasoning out what happens in your life? YES/NO
2. Does how the world works interest you? YES/NO
3. Do you like to understand how the underlying principles of things work? YES/NO
4. Do you see order and meaning in everyday life and things? YES/NO
5. Are you good at time management? YES/NO
6. Do you like quantifying? YES/NO
7. Do you see meaning in numbers? YES/NO
8. Do you like interpreting data and/or things? YES/NO
9. Do you like hypothesizing? YES/NO
10. Do you like planning? YES/NO

Score:

1. Count the number of yesses
2. Multiply by 10
3. Add percent sign

5. Kinesthetic/Sensory Module of Thinking

1. Do you need to experience something in order to make sense of it? YES/NO
2. Do you need to feel or touch or hold something in your hands in order to process it in your mind? YES/NO

3. Do you like to be shown how to do things instead of being told how to do things? YES/NO

4. Do you use lots of hand and/or body movements to get things across to people? YES/NO

5. Do you find that you raise your voice or your intonation changes when people don't seem to understand you? YES/NO

6. Do you need to get up and/or move in some way as you process information? YES/NO

7. Do you yawn a lot while focusing and thinking deeply? YES/NO

8. Do you have a good sense of timing when it comes to physical activities? YES/NO

9. Do you find it easy to participate in a group activity that involves a coordinated sequence of movements such as aerobics and dancing? YES/NO

10. Do you love movement and sport, even though you may or may not be proficient? YES/NO

Score:

1. Count the number of yesses
2. Multiply by 10
3. Add percent sign

6. *Musical/Intuition Module of Thinking*

1. Do you find yourself responding and even relying on your intuition as you process/digest information? YES/NO

2. Do you often find yourself referencing your gut instinct in conversation? YES/NO

3. Do you pick up on others' attitudes easily and correctly? YES/NO

4. Can you easily read between the lines? YES/NO

5. Can you easily feel the impact of toxic thinking in your mind and body? YES/NO

6. Do you find yourself intuitively predicting things? YES/NO

7. Are you a good judge of character? YES/NO

8. Do you instinctively feel when something is right or wrong? YES/NO

9. Do you find yourself not saying or doing something till it feels right? YES/NO

10. Do you feel yourself needing music in the learning environment? YES/NO

Score:

1. Count the number of yesses

2. Multiply by 10

3. Add percent sign

7. *Visual/Spatial/Imagination Module of Thinking*

1. Do you find yourself noticing color, light, depth, and shape around you? YES/NO

2. Do you notice mess and does it worry you? YES/NO

3. Do you notice things out of alignment like a picture hanging askew on a wall? YES/NO

4. Do you notice how well people are or aren't groomed? YES/NO

5. Do you need to express yourself artistically in drawing, painting, new theories, ideas, businesses, or any other form of creativity? YES/NO

6. Do you have lots of ideas swirling around your mind? YES/NO

7. Do you almost see literal "movies" in your head as you are listening to someone talking? YES/NO

8. Are you able to move furniture or rooms or physical things around in your head? YES/NO

9. Can you easily navigate your way through space, for example, when moving through apertures, moving a car through traffic, parking a car, and so on? YES/NO

10. Do you like and are you fairly good at producing various art forms such as illustrations, drawings, sketches, paintings, and sculpture? YES/NO

Score:

1. Count the number of yesses
2. Multiply by 10
3. Add percent sign

Once you have filled in your profile and worked out your scores, put them into Table III above.

Application Example

Look at the table below to see an example of how to apply the Gift Profile to your everyday life.

Table IV: Application Example

Digestion Stages	Module of Thinking	Describe Yourself
1. In order to focus I need to (conscious level):	Highest score: Intrapersonal 90%	I focus using Introspection at least 70–80% of the time. I find myself looking away as someone begins to talk to me in order to "go inside my own head" to focus.
2. In order to pay attention I need to (conscious level):	Second highest score: Visual/Spatial 80%	I pay attention by drawing pictures and doodling.

3/4/5. In order to analyze (consolidate/confirm/integrate) I need to (nonconscious level):	Third highest score: z Linguistic 75% Fourth highest score: z Kinesthetic 70% Fifth highest score: z Musical 60%	I analyze with words and intuition, and I feel something happening in my mind.
6. In order to apply I need to:	Sixth highest score: Interpersonal	I start asking questions or making comments.
7. In order to close I need to:	Seventh highest score: Logical/Mathematical	I start doing something in a logical, ordered way.

Fill in the table below with your gift profile. You can use Tables I and II above to help you. Feel free to use your own wording.

Table V: Your Application

Digestion Stages	Module of Thinking	Describe Yourself
1. In order to focus I need to (conscious level):	Highest score:	
2. In order to pay attention I need to (conscious level):	Second highest score:	
3/4/5. In order to analyze (consolidate/confirm/integrate) I need to (nonconscious level):	Third highest score: Fourth highest score: Fifth highest score:	
6. In order to apply I need to:	Sixth highest score:	
7. In order to close I need to:	Seventh highest score:	

How to Use Your Profile

Understanding your customized way of thinking allows you to be *you*. It enables you to work out strategies that maximize your ability to think, learn, and succeed in your unique way. It is the way to activate the power contained in the mindsets.

We can learn to adapt our environment to our needs. If you like wiggling or moving as you are focusing and paying attention, you can sit on an exercise ball rather than a stationary chair. You can even get a little ball for your seat that allows you to rock from side to side, which is easy to carry from room to room. You could use a stand-up desk with a supporting foot pad. Interestingly, the side-to-side or gentle rocking movement of a standing desk actually allows information to enter more effectively into your brain in the sequence used in your brain's wiring. A simple change can be revolutionary! I found these little changes made massive differences in the lives of my patients.

Even movement, to use the example above, is unique to each individual. Some people may move in a very obvious way; others may move in a way that is hardly perceptible. Some people who use movement to focus and pay attention will move at the beginning of a cycle of thought and then stop moving, and some people may analyze using movement. Using kinesthetic stimulation at the wrong point in your thinking cycle can frustrate your ability to learn and communicate, which is why it is so important to understand how we learn. When we understand our customized mode of thinking and how our brain is wired—that is, how we are designed to move through the world—we will learn more quickly, think more clearly, process information more quickly, accomplish more, and succeed!

Indeed, we can take every single "type A" personality on the planet and discover that each one of them has a different combination of the seven modules of thinking. We are more than a label or a test. It is our differences that make us who we are at our core. And it is in our differences that our customized thinking and resultant genius lie.

NINETEEN

Characteristics of the Seven Modules

What does each module of thinking look like in the real world? Below are several characteristics of each of the seven modules of thinking. You can use these descriptions to help you understand what your customized way of thinking will look like and also use them to add to and edit your Gift Profile. Some may apply, some may not, because these are just a sampling and not all-inclusive—these characteristics simply help you describe yourself.

Intrapersonal Module of Thinking

The Intrapersonal module of thinking includes deep thinking, decision making, putting things together, focusing, analyzing, and choosing. Intrapersonal thinking is, at its heart, the ability to stand outside of ourselves and analyze our own thinking. This is essentially the seat of our ability to choose, or our free will. We can analyze incoming and existing information, making decisions about what to think, say, and do.

This module of thinking is fundamental to introspection, self-knowledge, and understanding our own feelings, thoughts, and intuition. The ability to access our self-knowledge allows us to guide our behavior, understand our strengths and weaknesses, imagine concepts, plan activities, and solve problems. This module of thinking therefore incorporates self-discipline.

In sum, Intrapersonal thinking is:

- You are introspective and aware of your range of emotions.
- You have the ability to control and work with your thoughts and emotions.
- You are good at finding ways of expressing your thoughts.
- You are motivated to identify and pursue goals.
- You enjoy working independently.
- You are curious about the meaning of life.
- You can self-manage ongoing personal learning and growth.
- You attempt to understand inner experiences.
- You empower and encourage others.
- You desire solitude.
- You enjoy thinking strategies, journal writing, relaxing, and self-assessment strategies.
- You understand your limitations.
- You assess and evaluate situations.

Interpersonal Module of Thinking

The Interpersonal module of thinking involves social interaction, listening, sharing, building relationships, giving, and receiving love. Interpersonal thinking gives us the ability to understand and work with people.

This module of thinking incorporates sensitivity to and empathy with others, particularly for their moods, desires, motivations, feelings, and experiences. It allows us to respond appropriately to others as well and to read other people's moods—that is, to put oneself in another person's shoes. It enables us to pick up inconsistencies when listening to smooth talkers so we know whom to trust. It also refers to good managerial and mediating skills and the ability to motivate, lead, guide, and counsel others.

In sum, Interpersonal thinking is:

- You are a strong leader.
- You are good at networking.
- You can negotiate.
- You can teach.
- You enjoy bouncing ideas off other people.
- You love to talk.
- You like to organize.
- You happily mediate in disputes and are good at conflict resolution.
- You enjoy acting as a mentor to others.
- You have the ability to focus outward on other people.
- You sense other people's moods, temperaments, motivations, and intentions.
- You have the ability to influence others.
- You excel at group work, team efforts, and collaborative work.
- You bond with people.
- You form lasting social relationships.

Linguistic Module of Thinking

The Linguistic module of thinking deals with how you use language to express yourself. It also deals with your sensitivity to the meanings of words, sounds, rhythms, and different uses of language. This is expressed in different ways, such as being articulate or having the ability to think in words and use words effectively when you speak and/or write.

The domains that make up language, its structure and use, are:

Semantics: the meanings or connotations of words.

Phonology: the sounds of words and their interactions with each other.

Syntax: the rules governing the order in which words are used to create understandable sentences. One example is that a sentence must always have a verb.

Pragmatics: how language can be used to communicate effectively.

In sum, Linguistic thinking is:

- You express and explain yourself by writing and/or using lots of words.
- You like to argue, persuade, entertain, and instruct.
- You like to write, play with words, read, and tell stories.
- You have a good general knowledge.
- You ask a lot of questions.
- You like to lead and/or participate in discussions.
- You like storyboards, word processors, and voice recorders.
- You love reading and need lots of books around you.
- You spell well.
- You learn languages easily.
- You have a good memory for names, dates, and places.

Logical/Mathematical Module of Thinking

The Logical/Mathematical module of thinking deals with scientific reasoning, logic, and analysis. This type of thinking involves your capacity to understand the underlying principles of a connecting system, recognize logical and numerical patterns, handle long chains of reasoning in a precise manner, and manipulate numbers, quantities, and operations. This module also includes the ability to mentally calculate and process logical problems and equations, much like the types of problems most often found on multiple-choice, standardized tests.

The domains that make up logic and mathematics are:

Numbers: the ability to manipulate and use numbers effectively.

Pattern recognition: the ability to categorize, organize, and make associations in nature, numbers, words, stories, and life.

Identification: the attempt to find meaning in things.

In sum, Logical/Mathematical thinking is:

- You are intuitive and disciplined in your thinking.
- You like to calculate and quantify.
- You want to reason things out.
- You want to know what's coming up next.
- You love to roam in the realm of imaginary and irrational numbers.
- You find paradoxes challenging.
- You love to create theories of how things work.
- You like to work out and fully understand complex sequences.
- You need systematic proof of something before using it.
- You show the ability to recognize and then solve problems.

Kinesthetic Module of Thinking

The Kinesthetic module of thinking includes movement, somatic sensation, and moving around. Kinesthetic thinking helps you play soccer, run around, sit in a chair without falling off it, or navigate

153

your way down an aisle. This module of thinking includes integrating the sensations from inside your body as well. By definition, this is a very tactile, energetic, and multisensory type of thinking that involves the control of body movements, the ability to coordinate yourself, and the capacity to handle objects and things around you skillfully. It incorporates the need to touch, feel, and move things around, to maneuver or experience what is being learned.

In sum, Kinesthetic thinking is:

- You have good coordination.
- You show a good sense of timing.
- You approach problems physically.
- You explore your environment through touch and movement.
- You like to fiddle with and do things.
- You often stretch.
- You like role-play and drama.
- You love to dance.
- You need to move when thinking.
- You enjoy exercise.
- You enjoy crafts and hobbies.
- You demonstrate balance, dexterity, grace, and precision in physical tasks.
- You invent new approaches to physical skills.

Musical Module of Thinking

The Musical module of thinking might seem like it just involves the ability to sing or play a musical instrument, but, surprisingly, it also includes the ability to read patterns, identify rhythm, deal with instincts, and, most importantly, *read between the lines*. It works very extensively with the part of your brain called the insula, which is deep inside the Musical module of thinking and helps you to develop your instinct, allowing you to read between the lines in various situations.

Musical thinking allows you to sense meaning and verify it. For example, when you ask your friend, "Are you okay?" and she says, "Yes, I'm fine" (with a quiver in her voice), this module allows you to actually interpret that she's not fine. It's the ability to read people through their tone of voice and body language, rather than just listening to what they say.

This module of thinking incorporates sensitivity to pitch, melody, rhythm, and tune in sounds and movements, as well as the ability to produce rhythm, pitch, and forms of musical expression. It is also related to intuition, gut instinct, and reading body language. On one end of the human scale is the level of musical thinking attributed to interpretation of conversation, and on the other end of the scale is the level attributed to musical geniuses such as Mozart.

Some types of thought have a critical period for optimal development, and musical thinking is one of them. The years between the ages of four and six are the optimal time for developing sensitivity to sound and pitch. It is therefore during this time that musical ability is best developed. This does not mean, of course, that you will never be able to develop your ability beyond those years. All humans have the capacity to develop their musical thinking.

Music can help you learn. Classical music in particular has proven to be beneficial in classrooms and other learning environments.

In sum, Musical thinking is:

- You instinctively feel when things are right or wrong.
- You don't do things unless they "feel" right.
- You can't always explain why, but you know when someone is to be trusted or not to be trusted.
- You are highly sensitive to your surroundings and feel comfortable or uncomfortable in certain places.

- You are able to read between the lines of what people are saying.
- You find yourself interpreting the meaning behind things.
- You seek out sound.
- You respond to music.
- You like to compose music.
- You play an instrument.
- You can sing in tune.
- You keep time to music.
- You instinctively listen critically to music.
- You listen and respond to environmental sounds.
- You collect songs, instruments, and music.
- You create musical instruments.
- You use the vocabulary and notation of music.
- You hum often.
- You tend to tap your foot, finger, or pen when working or listening.
- You offer interpretations of the meaning of music.
- You have a highly developed intuition.

Visual/Spatial Module of Thinking

The Visual/Spatial module of thinking deals with the ability to see color, light, shape, and depth. You can close your eyes and use your imagination to see things that are not actually in front of your eyes; for example, you can imagine a loved one and call up a visual image from your nonconscious mind into your conscious mind. This is the ability to visualize in pictures and/or images, to see with the mind's eye, to make mental maps, to perceive the visual/spatial world accurately, and to act on initial perceptions.

156

Visual/Spatial thinking concerns internally representing the external, spatial world in your mind and being able to orient yourself in three-dimensional space with ease. Artists have high Visual/Spatial thinking, which expresses itself in great works of art like the masterpieces of Leonardo da Vinci and Michelangelo.

Yet this type of thinking is not restricted to the arts. Sir Isaac Newton and Albert Einstein, for example, expressed their high Visual/Spatial thinking in a more scientific manner.

This mode of thought is also not restricted to the physical sense of what something looks like. If this type of thought is high up in your sequence, then you build memory through abstract language and imagery.

Visually impaired people have very well-developed Visual/Spatial thinking, because they rely on what they see in their mind's eye.

In sum, Visual/Spatial thinking is:

- You often stare off into space while listening.
- You enjoy hands-on activities. That is, you learn by seeing and doing.
- You recognize faces but may not remember names.
- You navigate through spaces well; for example, you easily find your way through traffic.
- You think in pictures and visualize details easily.
- You perceive both obvious and subtle patterns and see things in different ways or from new angles. You are proficient in both representational and abstract design.

An Example of the Modules of Thought

Let us look at my profile. My highest score is Interpersonal. The first step in the sequence of thought (for everyone) is focusing.

So, if my highest score is Interpersonal, if I were in a classroom or boardroom I would concentrate best if I were focusing while interacting with the teacher or the people around me. I would better process information if I asked questions, because it would jumpstart my brain's sequence of processing incoming information. Working on my own, I actually "ask" a lot of questions about the material I am listening to or reading, often bombarding my husband, Mac, or my children with a million facts and questions!

On the other hand, if my highest score were Intrapersonal, I would most likely feel very frustrated if I had to ask people questions to focus. I would be concentrating deeply on the information I would need to understand; questions would interrupt my customized mode of thinking. When you determine the structure of your customized thinking, you can determine the triggers that allow you to maximize your brain function.

Remember, how high your score is for each of the modules simply determines how strong that trait is in your gift and its position in your cycle. If you have a really high score in one area, most likely those traits are very dominant aspects of your personality. For example, if I were to score in the seventies on the Interpersonal questionnaire, I most likely wouldn't need as much interaction during this step in the thinking sequence as I would need if my score were in the nineties. If your highest score was Intrapersonal, and you scored in the nineties, you most likely would need a lot of time at first to process information internally. If your score were in the seventies, you would need less time.

The most important part of understanding the structure of your gift is *freedom*. When you understand how you think, you will be free from any label—any label you have given yourself, any label the world has given you and, especially, any label you *think* the world has given you.

As you analyze your profile, remember that you cannot be put in a box. If Logical/Mathematical happens to be at the bottom of the order of your gifts, *it doesn't matter*. As you work on developing your mind through developing all seven modules, you enhance your cognition in multiple ways. I am thinking of one of my patients in my clinical practice back in South Africa who focused using his Musical thinking and paid attention through his Kinesthetic thinking. This student was failing math. He was, however, desperate to play a musical instrument, but his parents wouldn't allow him to do so until he improved his math grade. I profiled him and showed his parents that the way to improve his grades was to improve his focus, which for him was through his Musical thinking. We got him going on a keyboard, playing the drums, singing, and playing in a band. His thinking improved dramatically as a result; it wasn't long before his grades in *all* his subjects skyrocketed! The point is that if you can't focus and pay attention, you are not going to learn very well—nothing is going in to be learned!

Using your customized thinking can be tremendously rewarding. When you tap into how you think, you feel, *Wow! I'm actually quite smart. I understood that. I'm not so bad after all!* It's about the "Aha!" moments of life—we have all had those moments of excitement and satisfaction, and we should have them all the time.

When you suddenly feel so good because you have understood something, it is evidence that you are using your customized thinking; you have used your brain in the way it should be used. Grab that moment, grab that feeling, store it, frame it, and make sure you become consciously aware of that feeling. This is *you* at *your* best.

Indeed, your customized way of thinking operates a bit like dominoes. Imagine there are seven dominoes representing the seven modules of thinking. You push one, then the next one in line falls, and the next, and the next, and so on, in that particular order. Your order does not change with experience and maturity, but the interaction between the seven modules that make up your customized thinking get better with the development of your thinking, your wisdom.

Another Example of the Gift Profile

You may cycle through your customized thinking in this order:

1. Intrapersonal
2. Interpersonal
3. Linguistic
4. Visual/Spatial
5. Kinesthetic
6. Musical
7. Logical/Mathematical

Your thinking would involve a flow of electrical and chemical activity through the different parts of the brain in this order (see Image 18.1). This is a cycle of your thought.

Now, say we just changed 1 and 2, as in the example below:

1. Interpersonal
2. Intrapersonal
3. Linguistic
4. Visual/Spatial
5. Kinesthetic
6. Musical
7. Logical/Mathematical

This would produce a completely different type of thought pattern and a completely different perception of the world, because this is a completely different customized thinking pattern—a completely different way of thinking.

Essentially, there are an infinite number of thinking patterns, each giving rise to another thinking pattern or gift. Your customized thinking is not a static entity; the order stays the same, but you are a dynamic, thinking being, constantly developing and growing as you use your customized thinking—which means your intelligence *is in your hands*. As you think to understand, you are using your customized thinking, and this increases the branches and the networking capacity in your brain. These connections in the interlaced neural networks (thought clusters) increase the efficiency of the brain. The more you use your customized thinking, the more connections you make and the more efficient your brain becomes.

When you continually use your customized thinking, you can enhance and preserve the brain's powers as you move through life. The brain continues to change and grow into old age, making it an extremely unique organ both among biological and mechanical structures because it does not wear out. There is no expiration date on your potential!

Unique Combinations

In my own family, I see every day how each one of our unique combinations has a powerful impact on how we function. My husband, Mac, and I have four children. Although we all share many values and have a lot of things in common, it is our differences that make our life exciting as a family. We have reached the point of being able to recognize our differences as our strengths; we are at peace with thinking, speaking, and acting in different ways and trust one another unconditionally.

The gift concept helps us to see each other as different and unique. We understand that our differences are not a threat. It is liberating to realize that we do not have to compete with one another. Our differences facilitate community, which, as I discussed in the mindset section, is essential to success.

Customized Thinking and Purpose

To grow as a human being and to use our innate potential, we need to move away from what I call a "disability focus"—focusing on our weaknesses and forgetting about our strengths. We need to focus on what we can do, rather than what we think we can't do. When we do this, we will find that our customized thinking will naturally grow stronger. We need to stop desiring someone else's customized thinking and rather focus on and develop our own way of perceiving and understanding the world.

Unfortunately, one of the most concerning aspects in education today is the preoccupation with weakness. Students are often made to focus on what they cannot do and are not given the freedom to focus on their strengths. Educators and parents, most likely through no fault of their own, often do not take the time to discover what their students' strengths are. In many cases, they may not even acknowledge that some of their students have any strengths at all, especially if they happen not to be strong in Logical/Mathematical and Linguistic domains—the so-called school intelligences. And this is not limited to education; this applies in work and life as well.

The Gift Profile redirects our attention to our customized thinking. Rather than trying to categorize people, we can learn to recognize and celebrate their differences. Society as a whole can only progress if we understand that we don't all have to fit in one particular mold. Everyone has a role to play.

Indeed, we are *all* creative. We may have been taught that only those with a dominant Visual/Spatial or Musical thinking are creative, and we tend to see people as "creative" only if they happen to be artistic or musical in a conventional sense. Yet creativity is expressed through all the seven modules of thinking; we are being creative when we function within our customized thinking.

Few people would easily associate analytical thinking with being creative, yet there are many examples where it is extremely creative. The great Italian artist Leonardo da Vinci, for example, was clearly "creative." He left behind many masterpieces that attest to his prodigious talents. Yet he also had strong Logical/Mathematical thinking, which many educators would not easily attach to the idea of creativity. He designed the first helicopter, and he completed and recorded the first anatomical dissection. Albert Einstein is another example. He was clearly gifted mathematically and logically, yet he was certainly "creative." He may not have produced works of art like da Vinci, but he gave us many amazing insights into the universe. His ability to visualize the natural world was incredible. No one would ever describe Einstein as lacking in creativity!

Each one of us is a special part of this wonderfully unique puzzle that is life. To find our place in it, our purpose, we need to think in our own customized way. When we allow all seven types of our thinking to work together in their unique way, we begin to operate in our gift and move toward knowing, being, and accepting who we really are. We move away from trying to be what we are not; we stop trying to live up to other people's expectations; we quit feeling like we have to put up fronts or façades. We become someone who is able to

- Plan
- Strategize
- Imagine
- Listen
- Reason
- Guide
- Reflect
- Follow
- Evaluate
- Intellectualize
- Analyze
- Actualize
- Consider
- Create

And when we do all of the above well (at least most of the time!) we can become a great

- Leader
- Parent
- Follower
- Friend
- Educator
- Spouse
- Manager
- Professional
- Human
- Anything we want to be!

In other words, we will be a *success*!

Guidelines to Harness and Develop Your Gift

Below are several guidelines that will help you use and develop your different modes of thinking. The idea of this section is to focus on developing *all* seven modules of thinking, because all are needed for you to think properly in your customized way—that is, the way you use your modules, which is different from everyone else. Remember: we all use all seven modules of thinking, just differently. As humans we grow, change, and mature through life, which is reflected in the development of these seven modules of thinking. They are evolving as we evolve. So it's a great idea to develop and enhance each module as a part of your lifestyle, regardless of their order in your profile—which, remember, only shows how *you use* the modules and *not your skills* in mastering the modules. You are not trying to improve a weakness; you are developing and sharpening your customized thinking.

You enhance your Intrapersonal thinking when you:

- Develop your self-awareness by listening to and becoming aware of what you are thinking.
- Analyze your intuition when it has proven to be correct.
- Develop your senses, which increase your awareness.
- Have quiet time alone.
- Write down your dreams.
- Associate new and unique ideas with old ideas.
- See things from different points of view.
- Respond as fully as you can to aesthetically appealing objects.
- Solve problems and find solutions.
- Always see a situation as a challenge, no matter how bad, and find solutions to solve it.
- Are honest with yourself.
- Make the effort to listen deeply to others and to what they are really trying to say.
- Use the Switch On Your Brain 5-Step Learning Process.

You enhance your Interpersonal thinking when you:

- Do group work.
- Retell stories or tales.
- Use a thesaurus.
- Practice involving a group in your presentation or lesson and tuning in to others.
- Practice making people feel at ease in challenging situations.
- Spend time with people.
- Listen without interrupting and planning your own response.
- Listen twice as much as you talk.
- Put yourself in another's position and try to think how they think.

- Take a presentation skills course.
- Play "What if?" games.
- Take the time to coach or mentor others in something you are good at.
- Use the Switch On Your Brain 5-Step Learning Process.

You enhance your Linguistic thinking when you:

- Read, read, and read some more! This is the quickest and most effective way of building Linguistic thinking. Read a variety of literature, from the newspaper to novels, news magazines, and even comics. Read across a variety of different subjects.
- Increase your vocabulary by learning one new word a day. Within a year, you will have increased your vocabulary by 365 words. Practice using these words in different contexts.
- Apply effective reading techniques to improve your concentration and comprehension.
- Play word games like Trivial Pursuit, Scrabble, Cluedo, and General Knowledge.
- Do crossword puzzles.
- Learn a new language.
- Use the Switch On Your Brain 5-Step Learning Process.

You enhance your Logical/Mathematical thinking when you:

- Practice estimating.
- Practice remembering statistics, such as those for your favorite sports team.
- Become aware of how you use numbers automatically on a daily basis. For example, you calculate how much time is left till lunch or before work is over.
- Use numbers to rank, organize, and prioritize.

- Play mental calculation games. For example, if you are a passenger in a car, add up the numbers you see on license plates of other vehicles on the road.
- Use your calculator as a training device and not a crutch!
- Break apart information you want to remember.
- Play games that are an effective "mind sport," such as Backgammon, Chess, or Bridge.
- Make stories with numbers—let them talk to you.
- Memorize the telephone numbers of family and friends.
- Use the Switch On Your Brain 5-Step Learning Process.

You enhance your Kinesthetic thinking when you:

- Sit on a ball instead of a chair when learning.
- Stretch frequently.
- Do drama, including formal theater, role-playing, and simulations.
- Do creative movement, dance, and stretching routines.
- Engage in small manipulative tasks; for example, using flash cards and stamps.
- Make things.
- Play games such as scavenger hunts and Twister.
- Learn to play or make a musical instrument.
- Take up pottery or wood carving.
- Use the Switch On Your Brain 5-Step Learning Process.

You enhance your Musical thinking when you:

- Play classical music in the background when working.
- Have musical instruments (or make them) available and play them periodically.
- Do aerobic routines to music.

- Tap a rhythm with your feet in time to your fingers typing on the computer.
- Sing or hum while you work, even if it's under your breath so as not to disturb others.
- Read poetry.
- Pretend you are a disc jockey while you learn or work.
- Be aware of using inflection in your voice and notice the inflection in other people's voices.
- Make an effort to read body language.
- Listen to your intuition.
- Use the Switch On Your Brain 5-Step Learning Process.

You enhance your Visual/Spatial thinking when you:

- Read and create your own cartoons.
- Examine advertisements and billboards.
- Use poster displays in your office or class to help you think and express ideas.
- Work with flow charts.
- Use mnemonic systems, such as the Roman Room technique, body parts, numbers, and rhyme systems to remember, plan, and make up linked stories.
- Draw pictures or doodle when thinking.
- Practice differentiating between colors.
- Take an art course.
- Practice developing your visual memory by doing the da Vinci exercise—that is, stare at a complex object, memorize it, then close your eyes and try to recall it in as much detail as possible.
- Play imaginative games.
- Build complex LEGO structures.
- Take a robotics course.
- Use the Switch On Your Brain 5-Step Learning Process.

The Unique Mind and Unique Brain

Using science, we can consider how the mind impacts and changes the brain. If the brain is the physical substrate through which the mind works, and the place where our thoughts are stored and from which we speak and act, then each human brain is uniquely attuned to each person. Researchers from Binghamton University have even found they can identify different people from their different brain wave responses![1] Indeed, we even each have our own unique sense of smell, called an olfactory fingerprint.[2]

Our views of the world are reflected in the architecture of our brains.[3] From the macro level of the structure of each part of the brain, to the micro level of the neurons, to the subatomic level, to the quantum level of vibrations, we are all different. The basic genome is nearly the same in all of us, but it is utilized differently across the brain and body and among individuals. Even our proteins vibrate in different ways.[4]

Our customized way of thinking is expressed through our customized brain. This is what you have been discovering through the Gift Profile. In effect, your responses to certain stimuli such as movies, foods, celebrities, and words may seem trivial, but they say a lot about you because they are based on *how you think*—your customized gift. If we *mindfully* tune in to our ability to think and feel and choose—that is, this customized thinking—and choose to pay attention to our customized thinking and thoughts, we can understand how we think, the very core of who we are! Your thinking pervades all your choices, and it's a powerful uniqueness that you need to harness and use to your advantage.

In the next section, you will learn how to build memory that is useful and meaningful, memory that will help you succeed in gaining the knowledge you need to thrive in school, work, and life. You are going to *learn how to learn* in your customized and exclusive way!

The Switch On Your Brain 5-Step Learning Process

TWENTY

What Is Learning?

Why do I remember some things and forget others? Is there a way of improving my memory? How do I learn? How can I be *more* effective in my business meetings, at work, and in life in general? Does my memory just get worse as I get older? Can I prevent this from happening?

These are just some of the questions I get asked often. Indeed, who doesn't want to get smarter, improve their grades, or receive recognition at work? Over the past thirty years, I have found that to answer these questions involves an incredibly important aspect of mental self-care, which I called *beyond mindfulness* at the beginning of this book.

Mindfulness is the ability to bring attention to our self-awareness, to recognize how we are thinking or feeling at any one moment. It is a revolutionary step in changing the way we think and is becoming more and more popular in the Western world. Recent research has shown the manifold benefits of mindfulness, as well as voicing caution as to the robustness of the evidence base for the effectiveness of mindfulness alone.[1]

However, going *beyond* mindfulness means that you redirect the calm, organized, and insightful state gained from mindfulness into an extremely productive knowledge-gaining process, a process that enhances and cultivates the information you receive in a successful way for whatever purpose you need it. By using the five-step technique in this section, you will literally be using your mind to train your brain to grow effective and useful memory networks. Remember, mindfulness is step one; to go beyond mindfulness you need to go through four more steps to draw on your customized thinking (section 2) to activate the power of the mindsets (section 1). You will be firing up your mind to think, learn, and succeed!

Of course, going beyond mindfulness requires significant time and effort, which allow us to lead a life well-lived. Learning how to learn and build sustainable memory will not only get you where you want to go but also improve your mental and physical health. Yes—learning, hence effective memory building, has mental and physical health benefits! The bottom line: we have to remember *useful* memory in order to function successfully and have a healthy brain.

As I discussed in the mindset section at the beginning of this book, the technological revolution, notwithstanding its many benefits, has also impacted the way we think. It is almost as though many people have forgotten how to think deeply and intensely about knowledge. It is the "If I can google the information, why do I need to learn and remember it?" effect. An overreliance on computers and search engines is weakening people's focus, deep thinking, attention, and memory. Maria Wimber from the University of Birmingham, among others, has shown that long-term memory is not properly built when people passively and repeatedly look up information on their phone or computer. This habit will have a negative long-term effect on the mind and brain, even potentially setting us up for the dementias.[2] This increasing reliance on the internet is changing our thought processes for problem-solving memory and learning—we are supposed to be building memories in our brains, not on our phones. Researchers have found that "cognitive offloading," or the tendency to rely on things like the internet as an aide-mémoire, increases after each use.[3] Our connection to the web is affecting how we think to the point where people are less willing to rely on their knowledge and say they know something when they have access to the internet at the click of a button.

Digital platforms, therefore, have the potential to inhibit learning, retention, recall, and recognition of information. Hence, we literally have to learn how to use technology *properly* so as not to damage our mind and memory-building process. This process is critical to healthy brain function and success in school, work, and life.[4]

Because we merge with our environments, this is a significant problem that no amount of mindfulness alone will correct. We have to start at mindfulness but go beyond it to create new meaningful habituated memories, or we won't create sustainable and maintainable change in our lives.

Research indicates that as we grow more dependent on technology, so intellect weakens and toxic addictions rise. For example, the pull-down refresh action on smartphones is deliberately designed like a slot machine.[5] It changes our brain's reward system (much like drugs and the modern American diet), creating a desire to constantly refresh our phones. Even in brief conversations of ten minutes or less, the presence of smartphones hinders the development of a sense of intimacy, trust, and empathy, impacting our ability to form meaningful relationships.[6] Facebook's first president, Sean Parker, is, in fact, one of many in the tech industry who are currently concerned about these influences of the social media platforms they have been a part of creating.[7]

What Is Learning?

We need to make digital technology platforms work for us and not against us. We need to get our minds working properly again. Mental self-care incorporates understanding and using the power of mindsets by activating our customized thinking (see section 2), which, in turn, allows us to build the brain through learning to build useful memory. In this section, we will focus on building the brain through the Switch On Your Brain 5-Step Learning Process, a technique I researched and developed over thirty years ago.

I use the word *learning* throughout this book to indicate thinking and building useful memory with understanding. This is not rote learning or memory tricks. Healthy, productive learning is good, old-fashioned hard work that draws on the amazing capacity we have as humans to think and learn—the opposite of what the incorrect use of technology does.

We need to take responsibility for thinking and learning to succeed. No one is going to do it for us. We shouldn't be tempted to fall for the gadgets, gizmos, tricks, or DIY guides that promise to make us smarter and more intelligent overnight. Nothing will ever replace diligent, intentional, conscious, and corrective hard work. *Only mind activity will change the brain*, which will produce changes in what we say and do. This change requires diligence and discipline. The dangers of the current environment we live in have made us impatient, a trifle entitled, and mostly unwilling to sacrifice and work hard. And many schools are sadly reinforcing this through overuse of technology, neuromyths, and teaching to the test. Time and effort are honorable, time-proven ways to success.

Thoughts Are Real

When we learn, we are building thoughts. Thoughts occupy mental real estate. They are the neurobiological correlates of mind activity. Powerful technologies have established that these biophysical correlates of memory, which are called memory engrams, our thoughts, have real, solid, physical representation and are made of proteins.[8] These thoughts keep changing in response to our thinking; we essentially control our ability to build thoughts, and this building allows us to determine what our brains look like and what we want—and need—in our heads.

The physical representation of thoughts in the brain looks like trees but are actually clusters of neurons with dendrites. Dendrites hold the information of our minds and undergo changes (plasticity) during the moment-by-moment experiences of life. This is *learning in action*. These thoughts are necessary for the expression of memory and are the roots of what we say and do.[9] (See chapter 21 for the updated science of memory formation.) We cannot say or do anything without first building a thought, so whatever we say and do is first a thought that we built. Indeed, we are learning all day long and expressing these thoughts all day long. Learning is a part of being alive and consciously aware of life. Learning builds memories, and memories are used to express our mindsets, world-view, and, most importantly, our "youness."

Whatever you think about the most grows in your mind. What you choose to focus on will be imprinted into your brain, affecting what you say and do. In fact, what you say and do is a reflection of what is going on in your mind—a sobering thought! It is important to remember that what and how you are learning will either lead to success or failure. The power of the mind brings with it great responsibility.

Research indicates that the way we think—that is, the way we use our customized thinking—will determine whether we remember or forget information. How we think will determine whether we

Image 20.1

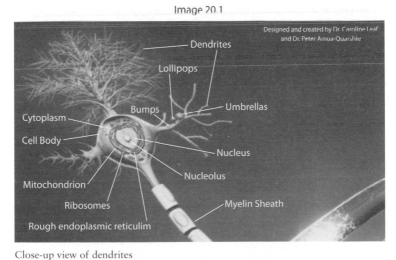

Close-up view of dendrites

build health or damage into our brains! If you want to remember successfully, you need to think in such a way as to involve your dendrites, the little branches on the top of neurons in the brain that resemble Christmas trees (see Image 20.1), and not just the synaptic connections between nerve cells (see Image 20.2). Chances are you may not have thought about memory or your thinking in terms of synapses and dendrites, but this is what you are about to discover in this chapter. Why? Because accurate thought-building leads to mind and brain health, which leads to success and happiness. Theories about how things work influence our mental health, lifestyles, education, and work. When we use our customized thinking, correct mindsets, and the technique in this section, we will build strong dendritic memories, which, trust me, are good for us!

Incorrect perceptions from incorrect theories about memory and learning (the neuromyths discussed earlier) will have a negative influence on how you perceive learning, which affects how you learn. In light of the fact that memory forms the core of your consciousness and the belief systems that make up *you*, correct perceptions of how memory works will also help you understand the importance of *thinking in your customized mode*. This is empowering because you will begin to see, through the lens of science, that you have *control over your memory and life* and can *always* change and improve. Understanding memory is a crucial part of your mental self-care regimen.

The Switch On Your Brain 5-Step Learning Process

My initial research focused on traumatic brain injury (TBI) and on people with learning disabilities, autism, chronic traumatic encephalopathy (CTE), and cerebral palsy, as well as those suffering from cognitive, communicative, and emotional pathologies and dementias.[10] The techniques I present in this section under the name of the Switch On Your Brain 5-Step Learning Process are the techniques I researched scientifically, developed, and used in my

Image 20.2

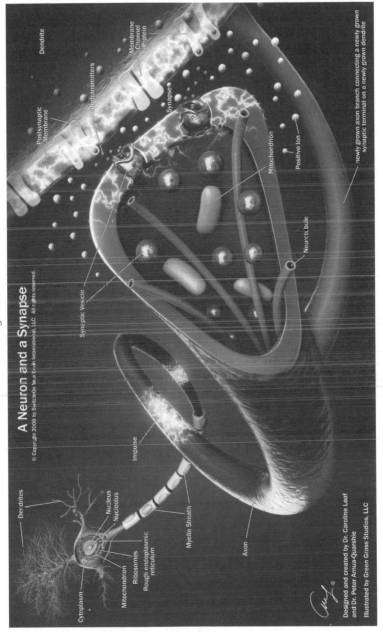

A Neuron and a Synapse

© Copyright 2008 by Switch On Your Brain International, LLC All rights reserved.

Dendrite

Membrane Channel Protein

Neurotransmitters

Synapse

Postsynaptic Membrane

Mitochondrion

Positive Ion

newly grown axon branch connecting a newly grown synaptic terminal on a newly grown dendrite

Neurotubule

Synaptic Vesicle

Impulse

Dendrites

Nucleus

Nucleolus

Cytoplasm

Mitochondrion

Ribosomes

Rough endoplasmic reticulum

Myelin Sheath

Axon

Designed and created by Dr. Caroline Leaf
and Dr. Peter Amua-Quarshie
Illustrated by Green Grass Studios, LLC

179

research and clinical practice and have been used successfully by hundreds of thousands of people around the world.[11] I observed positive incremental changes in academic, cognitive, intellectual, emotional, and social functioning among my patients when they used this program. And you can achieve the same!

It has been collectively demonstrated that just about every aspect of our thinking, learning, and intelligence—our brainpower—can be improved by intense, targeted, deliberate mind training. The Switch On Your Brain 5-Step Learning Process provides a technique for this kind of organized drive. Remember, with your mind you drive the brain in either an organized or disorganized direction—this is mind-directed neuroplasticity. Your mind can rebuild and restrengthen your memory, even when your brain has gone through the traumas of life. You can bring your brain under your control. You can improve your memory. You *can* succeed.

The Switch On Your Brain 5-Step Learning Process draws on an intersection of memory research, neuroscience, quantum biology, cognitive neuropsychology, language and communication, neuropsychology, psychoneuroimmunology, epigenetics, quantum physics, and intelligence research. It plays a vital role in the building of memory, which, as we have seen from the previous discussion, is the essence of the learning process.

The Five Steps to Successful Memory-Building

The Switch On Your Brain 5-Step Learning Process is made up of five important steps that facilitate this disciplined and directed learning process I have been discussing (see Image 20.3). These five steps will help you build memory and learn effectively using your customized way of thinking, which you learned about in the previous section.

Please be aware that this process will not work properly unless all five steps are used correctly. Each is designed to take you beyond short-term memory and into building *effective and useful*

Image 20.3

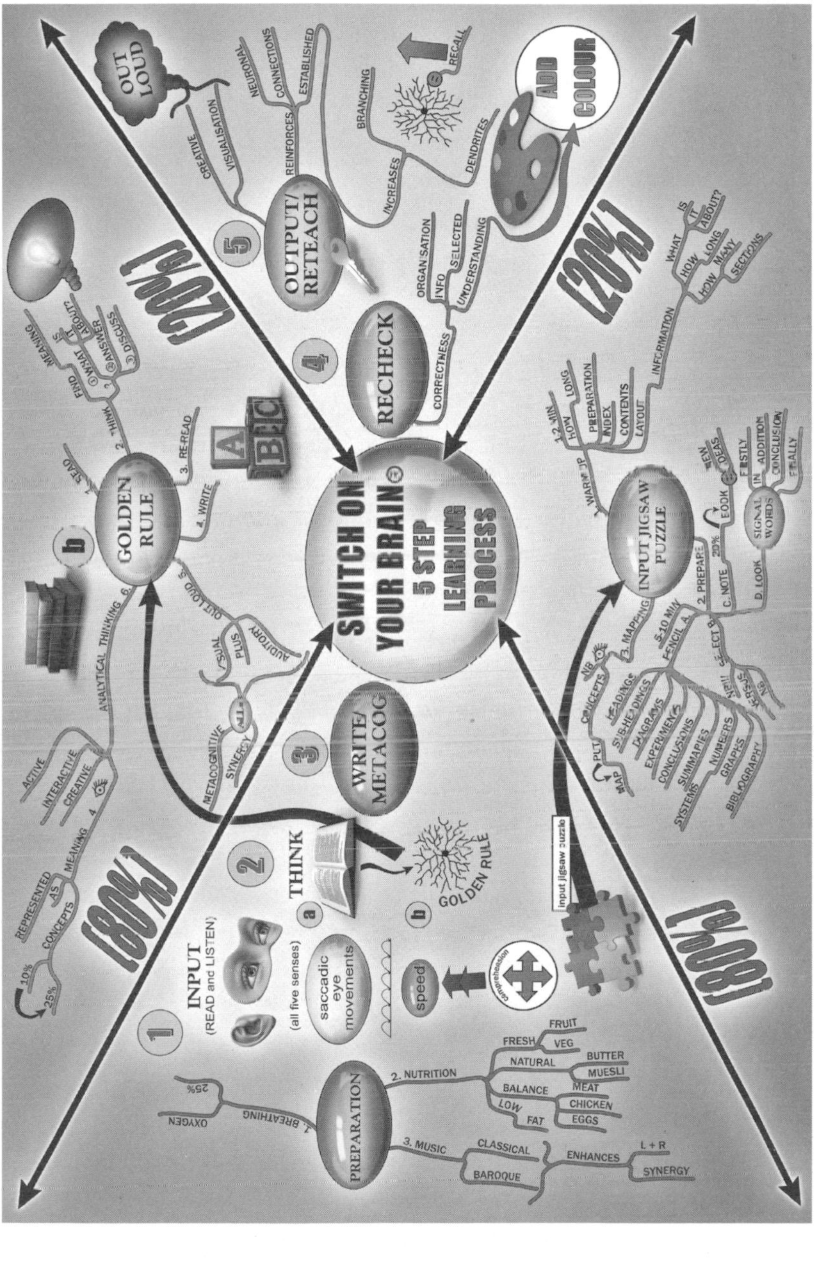

The Switch On Your Brain 5-Step Learning Process created by Dr. Caroline Leaf

long-term memory. Each is also designed to take advantage of a particular brain process, with all steps collectively moving toward the goal of memory building and learning. The five steps are:

1. **Input:** read, listen, watch
2. **Reflect:** ask, answer, discuss
3. **Write:** create the Metacog
4. **Recheck:** check for accuracy
5. **Output:** reteach

By using the Switch On Your Brain 5-Step Learning Process, you are activating your customized way of thinking to create useful memory. The focus becomes quality and not just quantity learning, because quantity without quality can actually damage the brain. Quantity plus quality engages the brain in a different way, producing a different kind of outcome. This is the kind of outcome that makes healthy, effective changes.

Indeed, operating *beyond mindfulness* adds a dimension of qualitative understanding and meaningfulness to the experience of life and learning that being aware in the now moment (meditation) and constantly relying on digital platforms does not. Not only are you gaining knowledge but you are bringing attention to your own experience of gaining knowledge. It is therefore productive *and* intellectually and meaningfully satisfying.

The easy-come, easy-go neuronal connections that come from lack of deep processing, rote learning, cramming for exams or meetings, and relying on digital platforms are quickly reversed. The Switch On Your Brain 5-Step Learning Process, on the other hand, maintains good thinking habits and creates memory banks of knowledge that can be used wisely. It requires deliberate, slow, steady work that forms new strong connections and dendritic arbors with lots of dendritic spines, a process that happens over cycles of about sixty-three days (see chapters 8 and 22). Each of the five steps is meticulously designed to stimulate the highest level of functional response in the brain in the most efficient way possible to guarantee great memories, contributing in turn to success in school, work, and life.

It is important to note that as knowledge is developing and skills are building in the nonconscious networks of your mind (see chapter 22), it is not uncommon to feel that you are not making progress. This is exactly why you must continue to plug away until the breakthrough comes. It's the old adage: good, old-fashioned hard work. Rote learning without understanding simply does not allow lasting memory to build, which is an integral part of success. In brain language (see more in chapter 21), shortcuts like reliance on technology or cram learning only generate computational activity in the cell bodies of neurons in brains, and will only build transient memories at the synaptic connections—not a good thing if you want to succeed. The persistence of sustained thinking, on the other hand, over about two months per chunk of information, solidifies the memory by constructing it into dendritic arbors, which are in effect like trillions of the most powerful quantum computers (see Image 20.1).

As I mentioned above, your thinking can change the structure of your brain, which is called *mind-directed* neuroplasticity and which I demonstrated through behavioral changes in my research. Dr. Carol Dweck, a Stanford University research psychologist, found similar results with math students.[12] Research from Harvard has shown that the mental practice that comes from thinking deeply until understanding is reached leads to actual physical changes in the brain—this ability of mere thought to alter the physical structure and function of our gray matter is powerful! The mental practice of thinking is so powerful that researchers have taught people to play the piano through their imagination as effectively as someone learning the traditional way—that is, with an actual piano![13]

One of the most exciting facts about the plastic brain is that the brain is never quite the same and is changing with every new piece of information we learn. This means that the brain can just keep getting better and better with mental practice, provided you are operating in your gift and building memory correctly. The systematic thinking-to-understand mental process captured within the Switch On Your Brain 5-Step Learning Process will forever change the way you learn and will stretch your potential to untold horizons. It will change your brain. It will change you and can be applied in all spheres of life!

Step 1: Input

The goal of input is straightforward: to understand what we are hearing, reading, and experiencing, and to get the information into the brain properly. Information enters the brain as a quantum signal through our senses and as an electromagnetic signal close to an area called the *entorhinal cortex* (see Image 20.4). The entorhinal cortex is responsible for the preprocessing of input signals (information) and is an important memory center in the brain.

Here's how you can ensure that information is properly entered in the Input process:

1. *Always read with a guide.* This is an instrument to guide your eyes while you are reading. This could be your finger, a pencil, or a pointer—not a ruler, folded piece of paper, or bookmark, as these block the text. A guide will improve your concentration span and your comprehension by about 50 percent because it uses both sides of the brain at the same time. If you don't read with a guide, your concentration span will be shorter. You will think you are tired when you are not, because you are not using both sides of the brain at the same time, working in harmony.

2. *Read out loud.* Do this wherever and whenever possible, which obviously depends on your immediate circumstances. You need to see *and hear* the words you are reading. This auditory stimulation dramatically increases the possibility of understanding and decreases the chances of making mistakes in understanding the information being read. It also increases self-regulation, allowing your gift to operate at optimum levels.

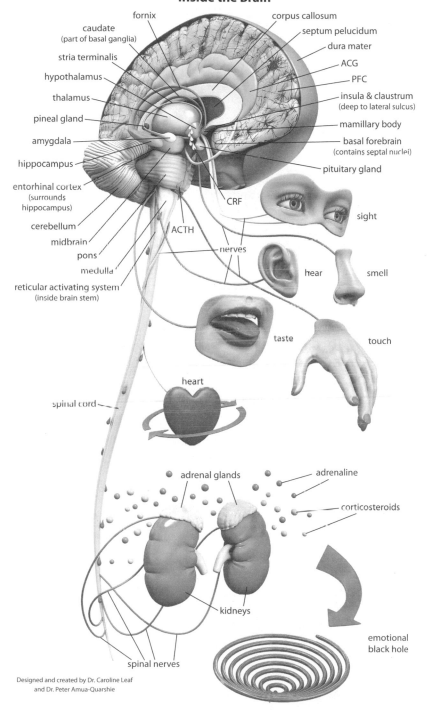

Image 20.4
Inside the Brain

fornix
caudate (part of basal ganglia)
stria terminalis
hypothalamus
thalamus
pineal gland
amygdala
hippocampus
entorhinal cortex (surrounds hippocampus)
cerebellum
midbrain
pons
medulla
reticular activating system (inside brain stem)

corpus callosum
septum pelucidum
dura mater
ACG
PFC
insula & claustrum (deep to lateral sulcus)
mamillary body
basal forebrain (contains septal nuclei)
pituitary gland

CRF
ACTH
nerves
sight
hear
smell
taste
touch
heart

spinal cord

adrenal glands
adrenaline
corticosteroids
kidneys
spinal nerves
emotional black hole

Designed and created by Dr. Caroline Leaf and Dr. Peter Amua-Quarshie

3. *Read a chunk of information at a time.* A chunk is between one to three sentences long, a bite-sized amount of information. We cannot build memory properly when we read through a large section of work at once and try to memorize it. This kind of reading leads to a level of understanding but does not build long-term memory. However, easily digestible amounts of information, bite-sized chunks, will lead to understanding. As when you eat bites of food, you are digesting small amounts of information at a time. You can do a quick read-through of the whole piece of information first, then come back and reread chunk by chunk to get those dendrites building.

4. *Have the right attitude about what you read* (review section 1 on mindsets). A wrong mindset affects the quantum and electrochemical reactions in the brain, which, in turn, will affect your understanding of what you are reading, slowing you down. Be as interactive with the material as you can. Visualize whatever it is you are about to read, whether a book, notes, or an article, as having been written by a person who is telling you something. Ask yourself what that person is trying to tell you in order to understand the meaning of what you are reading. Interact with words on the page as if you are interacting with whoever wrote them. To get into the habit of interacting with what you learn, ask yourself about the information, answer yourself by paraphrasing what you have read, and discuss it with yourself. This interaction allows the nerve cells to switch on the gene that makes strong long-term memories grow in the dendritic branches.

5. *Listen carefully!* When listening, listen with a pen and paper and interactive thoughts. Here is how to listen attentively and intently to build good memories:

- Write down something—words, sentences, drawings. Writing while listening is the important process here. This allows for deeper mental activity, which prevents your mind from wandering off. This also helps you order your mind.

- Get as interactive as you can. Ask questions, either out loud or silently, and repeat phrases the speaker is saying (silently to yourself, obviously) to mentally discuss the topic.
- Control and discipline your thought life. There will be many intruding thoughts that are just there or that get stimulated by the information you are receiving. Acknowledge them, but don't indulge them until you have all the information you need from the person speaking.

What Is Happening in the Brain

To give you an idea of how your brain responds to your mind-in-action, below is a simplified explanation. Use Image 20.4 to help you follow this analysis. (See chapter 21 for more information on synaptic connections, cell bodies, dendrites, and the quantum action of how memory forms.)

As you input information into the brain by listening and reading and experiencing through your five senses, the information passes through the brain on two levels: on a quantum level as a cloud of particles in superposition, and on an electromagnetic and chemical level flowing through areas in the brain in a sequence, which is very different and much slower than the quantum activity. The electromagnetic and chemical flow appears to go from the entorhinal cortex (like a doorway), to the thalamus (like a satellite station), to the cortex (the outer part of the brain), where long-term memories are stored and existing memories get activated. Your emotional state, which results from the activation of these memories, stimulates the hypothalamus, which quickens the release of chemicals to help with memory building. It is important to stay calm while in this process, because anxiety will block effective memory building. From this point, the information flows into the amygdala (like a library of emotional perceptions), where more preparation for memory building is done, and finally into the hippocampus, the structure where short-term memory is built and then converted to long-term memory and stored in the outer cortex over twenty-one days. This flow of electrical activity moves backward and forward in a looping way between all these structures as the memory is starting to form, while the quantum activity occurs across the entire brain. A lot is happening as you read and listen!

As you go through this step, it is important to remember that we are thinking beings; we think all day long. Thinking builds thoughts, and thoughts occupy physical, mental real estate in the brain. Thinking properly will produce understanding and build good thoughts (which are the same thing as memories). Conversely, toxic thinking, whether it is on an emotional level or through shallow thinking habits, can make the brain toxic and affect our ability to learn.

Step 2: Focused Thinking/Reflect

The aim of this step is to teach you how to think properly, and, in doing so, develop your phenomenal capacity to build effective, long-term memory into your dendrites. The Golden Rule of the Switch On Your Brain 5-Step Learning Process is to *think to understand* the information you are trying to remember. Thinking to understand involves three steps: asking, answering, and discussing.

For the Focused Thinking step:

1. *Read* a chunk of information—between one to three sentences—out loud, with your guide (pencil, pointer, or finger).
2. Stop and *ask* yourself what you have read.
3. Now, *answer* yourself by looking at what you have just read. Then answer yourself by rereading the chunk of information out loud and circling the concepts. Don't underline or highlight words. Those are passive actions, because they don't require you to think, analyze, or understand what you have underlined or highlighted. Circling is active.

4. Next, *discuss* this chunk of information with yourself, still looking at the sentence(s) you have just read. Discussion means you explain it to yourself over and over in your own words until you understand. If you can't work out what it means, ask someone or make a note to find out later.

5. As you are discussing, check how much you have *circled*. If it is more than 40 percent of a page, you have circled too much and probably don't understand yet. Go back and reread and rediscuss until you can reduce what you have circled down to 15 to 35 percent of the content. If you have circled more, you were probably thinking that if you select lots of words, you would remember more. Let me assure you, the opposite will happen. If you focus on too many words, you will make your memory worse, not better. It is between 15 and 35 percent of the sentences that contain the most important concepts; the rest of the sentences are filler words and don't need to be written down. Once you feel you have fully understood the concepts of the chunk you have just read, you are ready to write them down (step 3).

What Is Happening in the Brain

The Focused Thinking step challenges the brain to move into a higher gear, which is what it is designed for: deep, intellectual thought! If your mindset is right (see section 1), a level of expectancy builds and chemicals are released during this level that allow deep learning to occur. For example, dopamine and endorphins are released as your understanding is developing, which help you learn effectively and encourage you to keep learning.

On a cellular level, the dendrites become involved in the process of learning. Great memories are beginning to form (see the detailed discussion in chapter 21).

On a structural level, the whole brain is involved when you think, with waves of extra activity in different parts of the brain.

The corpus callosum is activated as you integrate information. The hippocampus is activated to convert the information from short-term memory to long-term memory and store it in dendrites in the cortex. The frontal lobe is responding to your decision making and planning. The neurons are responding by growing dendrites to store the information. Integration across the left and right sides of the brain occurs.

Step 3: Writing/Metacog

The Writing step involves writing the information down that you selected during the analytical Focused Thinking step. I recommend you use the "brain friendly" way of writing I have created, called the Metacog. This way of writing down information looks like the branching of dendrites on neurons (see Image 20.1). Dendrites have an arbor-like structure and look like trees with many branches. Their pattern and shape are dictated by the pattern and shape of the neural network of the memory you are building as you ask/answer and discuss your way through the information.

It is really important to write concepts down through the ask/answer/discuss process, because this reinforces healthy dendrite growth and really forces you to think about your thinking. The brain operates like a quantum computer, and deep-thinking mind action provides the signal to the quantum computer. As you think (step 2 = ask/answer/discuss), you create signals in your brain; as you write words down in the Metacog brain-friendly format, you reinforce and strengthen the quantum signals and what you have just grown in the dendrites. You are literally influencing your genetic expression and growing your brain at will!

It is interesting to note that just by looking at a Metacog (see the appendix for examples), you stimulate your brain to process information from detail to big picture and big picture to detail, which helps to consolidate strong memory across the left and right hemispheres of the brain. The Metacog is the visual tool of the Switch On Your Brain 5-Step Learning Process and is a mind-friendly way of writing that looks like the branching of a tree and its leaves. Its pattern and shape are dictated by the pattern and shape of the actual network being built as a person thinks. Making a Metacog is almost like looking inside your brain to gain insight into your mind; it is like putting your mind and brain on paper! The Metacog is a great way of getting your creative and memory juices flowing. It's also very insightful, and you will see things you didn't see before as well as think on a much deeper level. The Metacog literally changes you into a person of meaning living the good life!

Everyone can think and learn, and the Switch On Your Brain 5-Step Learning Process, as a neuroplasticity-driven system, stimulates the natural design of the brain, which is intentional deep thinking, resulting in understanding and strong, useful memory.

Through this process, the skills necessary to become an innovative, lifelong learner can be mastered. As such, this process is at the cutting edge of brain and learning research because it teaches people how to think, learn, and manage knowledge.

How to Create a Metacog

Did you know that every time you read a sentence, your nonconscious mind doesn't select every word to build a memory? You naturally and instinctively try to work out its meaning, which is the essential 15 to 35 percent of concepts per sentence. These concepts, or essential information, are what you will end up writing down on your Metacog. If you use more than that, you will have too many words to work with, and this redundancy will interfere with the memory of what is important. Between 15 and 35 percent is our ideal amount of information, because less than 15 percent will cause gaps in your memory and more than 35 percent can interfere with memory retrieval.

191

Following the principles of creating a Metacog in the correct sequence, every single time, is an important part of successful learning. Below are the instructions for building a Metacog.

1. *Preferably on a blank piece of paper, write the name of what you are working on in the center of your page.* This could be the chapter or section of work you are studying; it could be the meeting you are about to attend; it could be an article you are reading and want to remember; it could be a holiday you are planning; it could be a blog post or an essay you are planning to write.

2. *Try to print all the words you put onto a Metacog.* Don't write in cursive script. It is easier to remember something that is printed. Write the main categories in capital letters so they stand out. Write details lowercase.

3. *Each concept word must be on its own line.* You literally build a sentence on branched lines, one word per line. You have to decide on logical, propositional relationships between the concepts you select. This relationship needs to be reflected structurally on the Metacog, which is why you need only one word or concept on a line. Words on linked/connected lines lead to a spreading activation in which each concept triggers the next one in a logical and meaningfully associated way. This is what is happening inside your brain. More than one concept on a line interferes with the correct structuring of a Metacog and turns it into a type of flow diagram or a linear summary. This is fine once you have mastered the concepts, but not while you are mastering them. You need to build and create to learn. Each concept has its own electrical representation in the brain. If you put two words on a line, it is the same as putting two electrical representations onto a dendrite; the two collapse into one and half the meaning can be lost and/or confused.

4. *Put the first subheading on a branch that radiates out of the central bubble.*

5. *Write the rest of the information in concept form—the 15 to 35 percent (don't write out full sentences!)—radiating outward*

in branched format from that subheading. You should have lines branching from the subheading; write the words on these lines, which are much like branches of a tree. Remember to put one word per line as in point 3 above.

6. *The information radiating from the subheadings should progress from general to more specific.* This means that you "grow" branches outward from the main category to accommodate the 15 to 35 percent you have selected.

7. *These concepts must be written on the line, not next to the line or under the line.*

8. *Once you have selected and written down everything about that subheading, go to the next one and repeat the process until the whole section of work has been written onto the Metacog.* You are essentially doing the first three steps of the Switch On Your Brain 5-Step Learning Process together—so, Input, Think, and Write for one chunk of information, then Input, Think, Write for the next chunk of information, and so on.

9. *The shape of the branches you are growing on your Metacog is, in a sense, matching the branches you are growing in your brain on the dendrites.* The dendritic arbor in your brain is being reflected as a branched Metacog on paper. Without your being consciously aware of it, your neural network will dictate the shape of the branches on your Metacog. That's why I like to say that a Metacog is your "brain on paper." It's as though, as you draw the Metacog, your brain has already created the same pattern as a memory. If the words are all over the page, and not on logically connected lines, that's what will happen to the storage of information in your brain. It will be all over the place, and you won't be able to access the information when you need it.

10. *Start your Metacog in the top right-hand corner of the circle and work clockwise from left to right. You can go counterclockwise if it is easier or if you are left-handed.* As we mostly work from left to right, the Metacog generally follows the same format. You will need to rotate the page as you go so that you always work from

left to right. In doing this, you will find that half the Metacog is upside down. This is actually a good thing, because as you rotate the page, you will promote synergy between the two sides of the brain. This turning of the page will also keep you awake and alert. It isn't wrong if you prefer to read your Metacog without turning it, but brain research shows that this crossing over is good for deep thinking. You may actually also find that it is more natural to rotate your page as you instinctively work from left to right.

11. *Remember to always apply the Golden Rule of the Switch On Your Brain 5-Step Learning Process to understand how and when you select concepts: ask, answer, and discuss.* This is the conversation you need to have with yourself, as you read in the Think step. You only want between 15 and 35 percent of information to go down on your Metacog to make sure you retain the essentials; you need to think about and understand what you are reading. You are not just trying to summarize information. You are filtering out what is superfluous and keeping only the relevant information.

12. *Use color simply to enhance organization at the Recheck phase (step 4) if you want to, but only after you have written down everything you think is important.* Your Metacog will be more visually appealing with color, but you do not have to use it. When you first make your Metacog, use one color—for example, a lead pencil—so you do not interrupt the flow of thought in your brain. It also makes it easier to erase if you make mistakes, so you don't have to redo your Metacog altogether. Only add color in the Recheck phase, as a self-monitoring and memory-enhancing tool, if it helps you.

13. *This step is entirely optional: use pictures, symbols, shapes, and images supportively to help with memory if, and only if, it comes naturally.* You do not have to create an image for every word but rather for groups of concepts. As in the use of color, it is better to put the pictures onto the Metacog in the Recheck phase (step 4). When you concentrate on understanding and selecting

15 to 35 percent of the content, a picture may come to mind. If it does, you can put it on the Metacog. However, don't spend too long trying to create a superb image at the expense of concept selection. It's important to do what comes naturally to you. There will be plenty of time to add pictures (the simpler the better) in the Recheck and Output steps. Pictures are helpful to activate the nonconscious levels of learning, where metacognition is a strong driving force behind our conscious thinking. However, the use of pictures and whether you use them at all, like everything else, will depend on your gift—your default mode of thinking.

14. *Remember you build a Metacog, which means you are building a memory into dendrites.*

15. *There are various apps that you can use to build Metacogs on your computer, and even though I use some of these, I only use them once I have mastered the content by a hand-drawn Metacog.*

What Is Happening in the Brain

As you use a Metacog, the frontal lobe, parietal lobe, temporal lobe, and occipital lobe of your brain all work together to integrate and apply the information. More neurotransmitters (serotonin, dopamine, norepinephrine, and acetylcholine glutamate) are released from the brainstem and travel up through the limbic system (in the middle of the brain) into the cortex where the memory trees—the neurons—are found. The prefrontal cortex (PFC)—the outer front part of the frontal lobe—becomes very active and keeps the information active in the neurons "in mind," monitoring and manipulating the contents of your short-term memory. The PFC works with other areas in the frontal lobe and the other lobes of the brain to make decisions, shift between the different bits of information, analyze, and so on. Quantum information is active across the entire brain. A positive attitude ensures that genes are switched on for protein synthesis and good memories can form. (See the detailed discussion in chapter 21 about synaptic connections, cell bodies, dendrites, and the quantum action of how memory forms over sixty-three days.)

Creating Metacogs can work for anyone and everyone. They go much further than summarizing, notetaking, or brainstorming. They allow you to extract, store, and later recall 100 percent of the information you need for tests, exams, presentations, and the application of skills. They literally force you, by their very nature, to think deeply and intensely in a deliberate and self-reflective way.

As I mentioned above, when you are deliberately intentional about your learning, the two sides of your brain work together at the same time, creating a different depth of processing that leads to success in school, work, and life.

English is not the only language to embrace a linear script—straight lines in written form. Linear script can be from left to right, right to left, or even up and down. However, reading from the center outward is moving from big picture to detail, and that is your right hemisphere's way of processing. Your eyes will also read from the outer branches inward toward the center, moving from detail to big picture. That is your left hemisphere's way of processing. This act of creating a Metacog stimulates the corpus callosum to perform its natural function; that is, to get both sides of the brain working together integrating information across the hemispheres. The Metacog is essentially a tool that facilitates the switch to useful and meaningful long-term memory.

In earlier sections you learned that the raw material of consciousness is made up of neurons (nerve cells with a cell body), an axon, and dendrites. When you listen, see, talk, or learn, all this information goes into your brain as electrical and quantum activity. The more you stimulate your brain, the more you grow dendrites and, hence, useful and meaningful long-term memory. When you use a Metacog, you facilitate dendrites to grow in an organized, linked way, across both sides of the brain. The denser, more organized dendritic growth there is in your brain, the more intelligent you become and the more successful you will be.

Yet it is important to note that your Metacog will look *very different* from other people's Metacogs because everyone has a different gift—or customized mode of thinking. Your Metacog may be neat. Another person's may be messy. Yours may have lots of colors. Someone else's may have none. You may use more words. Someone else's may have fewer words.

Often, people mistakenly think that you have to be visually oriented to create a Metacog and learn from it, but this is not the case. You will create a Metacog according to your customized mode of thinking, so your Metacog is, in essence, customized to you. A Metacog is useful for *everyone* because it's a tool that allows your mind to work at optimum levels.

Step 4: Recheck/Revisit

Recheck is the fourth step of the Switch On Your Brain 5-Step Learning Process. This is the next important step that contributes to the building of useful long-term memory into the dendrites.

It's a very simple yet extremely powerful process. All you have to do is deliberately and intentionally go through your Metacog to see if it makes sense and if it has all the necessary required information on it. It goes without saying that you can't learn from something that doesn't make sense to you. The Recheck process is a cross-evaluation of the content of your Metacog.

For the Recheck step:

1. Make sure you understand the Metacog you have made.
2. Make certain you are happy with the information you have selected, which will be in concept form.
3. Look for whether you have too much or too little information.
4. Ask yourself if the Metacog makes sense, and if it doesn't, edit till it does.
5. Check whether you have organized the information in a logically associated way.

6. Check for cross-linking of information.

7. Check if you can make the concepts easier to remember by adding more pictures, symbols, or colors, or maybe even deleting some words or images.

At this point in the Switch On Your Brain 5-Step Learning Process you will have stored information effectively enough, provided you have properly followed the process, to be able to access it later wherever and whenever needed and to retain at least 60 to 90 percent—even 100 percent—of the information. To do even better, you need to move on to the final step of the Switch On Your Brain 5-Step Learning Process.

What Is Happening in the Brain

The Recheck/Revisit stage allows you to consolidate and reinforce memory of your work. It will soon become apparent if you have not fully understood what you are trying to remember. You will also gain insight into the work and see things you didn't see before if you do this step properly.

At this stage, you will have gone through whatever you are working on four times already, and will be about to go through it for the fifth time, probably without even being aware that you have gone over it so many times. This repetition is excellent because it activates quantum activity across the whole brain. (See the detailed discussion in chapter 21 about synaptic connections, cell bodies, dendrites, and the quantum action of how memory forms.)

Step 5: Output/Reteach

Output/Reteach is the final step of the Switch On Your Brain 5-Step Learning Process. In this step, you need to play "teacher" and sequentially reteach all the information that is on your Metacog.

Teach it to your dog, your cat, or whoever will or won't listen to you! You can even reteach yourself in the mirror.

Explain what you are learning out loud. Using all your senses will make your brain work harder, and your memory will be more effective as a result. Once you are happy with the reteaching of your Metacog, then it is essential to test yourself in some way. You can create some questions you think may be asked by your boss or teacher. Ask yourself questions that will help you apply the information to the life skill you are developing.

The mental practice that happens in this Output stage strengthens existing new dendrites and increases the spines on the outside of the dendrites, which is a good thing.

How to do the Output step:

1. Since this is the step where you reteach yourself, stick your Metacog up somewhere.

2. Teach it to someone or something—even to a pet, or to yourself in the mirror. If you don't have another living being handy, you can even teach your pencil!

3. Reteach in the way that you would like to have had the information explained to you or as though you are explaining to people in a second language. This involves explaining what you have learned carefully in multiple ways and in detail, and elaborating by way of extra examples.

4. The Output/Reteach step involves imagining and seeing as though watching a movie of exactly what it is you are learning. Paint a picture in your mind of the information on the Metacog. In other words, make the information on your Metacog come alive. Use your imagination—research has shown that imagination leads to great physical changes in the memory.

5. Continue reteaching until you can answer difficult questions without even looking at the Metacog.

6. You will normally have to go through the Metacog at least three times before you can confidently teach with full understanding, better than your teacher or lecturer or boss.

   It is at this point that you are ready to go into the test or examination, give the presentation, run the meeting, or solve a problem, with or without looking at the Metacog.

7. If you find while reteaching that something is not clear on your Metacog, then this is the time to look back at your notes or text and fix it up.

8. Look for trigger words, phrases, or images that bring back whole chunks of information into your mind.

9. This step should be done two to three days before a test, exam, or presentation. Before the test, you should go through the previous three steps daily or weekly, working through sections of information and making your Metacogs.

What Is Happening in the Brain

The Output/Reteach step also creates new connections. During this step, the new memories are consolidated, confirmed, and integrated with other memories. New connections are made, leading to the ability to apply the information in multiple ways.

The harder you think, the more dendrites you grow, and the more connections form between the dendrites via the dendritic spines. Useful knowledge is not just the storing of information but the ability to link and integrate it with other information and apply it.

The Switch On Your Brain 5-Step Learning Process achieves this because each step is designed to build strong, connected, and useful memories. The slow, steady work of the Switch On Your Brain 5-Step Learning Process ensures that accuracy and consolidation have occurred in the neural networks, specifically the dendrites. The entire brain is challenged to work as an integrated whole, creating good communication within the specific memory formed in the dendrites, as well as among the neural circuits. This increases the flexibility of thought.

The Timing of the Switch On Your Brain 5-Step Learning Process

In effect, there are three levels of thinking that are happening in this process. Level one, the Input step, stimulates thoughts that are just fleeting, which will disappear very quickly, within twenty-four to forty-eight hours, if not sooner, if they aren't captured in some way.[14] Level two, therefore, involves more deliberate thinking to capture those thoughts, which is the Focused Thinking/Reflect step. As you are asking/answering and discussing, you are literally "capturing and feeding" the memory. To keep the memory growing, you need to move through all five steps of the process in the same session (which can be from forty-five to sixty minutes) to really pin the concepts down and start moving them toward becoming a useful and meaningful long-term memory. Remember, the Writing/ Metacog step 3 is where the selected concepts are written onto a Metacog, the Recheck/Revisit step 4 is where the concepts are checked for accuracy and insight, and the Output/Reteach step 5 is where you explain and teach what you have just begun to master. Most times steps 1 and 3 are done together and steps 4 and 5 are done during final prepping for an exam, presentation, and so on.

The third level of thinking involves consistently, deliberately, and intentionally using the five steps daily for at least three consecutive weeks. You will literally cycle through the five steps multiple times in one forty-five to sixty-minute session, building understanding layer upon layer. You then repeat the twenty-one-day cycles as often as is needed to automatize the information so it's always available. Research shows that at least two more cycles of twenty-one days are needed, so plan on at least another forty-two days (or sixty-three days total) when preparing for an exam or to master a new concept.

Applications of the Switch On Your Brain 5-Step Learning Process

What does this look like if you are at school and preparing for an exam? It means you start learning each day as you get new information in class. So, the five-step process becomes how you master what you learned that day—both in the classroom as a note-making technique, and at home doing homework. This means you are building Metacogs consistently, and, by the time tests and exams come along, you only have to add on the new information and literally do rechecks in preparation! This is what I trained my patients to do, whether it was to build their brain after a brain injury, deal with a learning problem or emotional issue, or purely to improve academics. It was such a powerful tool in my practice, and my research showed up to 75 percent improvement in academic, cognitive, social, emotional, and intellectual function. In some cases, I had an almost 200 percent improvement. The process is so profoundly efficient that my patients were pleasantly surprised every time. Hundreds of thousands around the world are using these techniques now. The carryover into life and the long-term is also profound because your brain literally becomes retrained with the discipline of the five steps, so you start applying it in everything as a way of thinking about everything. It changes your intelligence, and wisdom becomes observable in every sphere.

I have also trained thousands of teachers, as I mentioned earlier, to use the Switch On Your Brain 5-Step Learning Process as a way of delivering information to students to stimulate deep thinking and learning—so their lessons are taught in the framework of the five-step process. Some schools have even put their entire curriculum into Metacogs. I would organize their curriculum in three-week cycles to take advantage of the way memory builds.

If you have already left school or university and are part of the working world, you may wonder whether the Switch On Your Brain 5-Step Learning Process will have any value for you at all. It certainly does. Today, more than ever before, there are no limits to what you can achieve, especially when equipped with the right tools.

This applies in and out of school and in business, since knowledge management, as mentioned in the introduction, has become so crucial a challenge to adding much-needed value and meaning in the workplace. The very competitive nature of the twenty-first-century workplace demands companies be constantly more efficient at processing information. The Switch On Your Brain 5-Step Learning Process meets this need, allowing you and your teams to switch on your brains to ever higher levels. On a corporate level, there are many applications. I have had CEOs of huge companies using the five steps and building Metacogs of the endless documents they need to read and understand to present or discuss in a board meeting. They are excellent as a presentation and discussion tool in a meeting. A Metacog is a particularly powerful tool to use when you are trying to understand or work out something and remember the information, because, through the five steps, you have to really think deeply to find the 15 to 35 percent to write down as compared to the shallower thinking used when you write down every word.

The five steps, with the third-step Metacog, are also a great note-taking tool in meetings and lectures. A great way to practice getting efficient at this is to Metacog while watching the news or a lecture on YouTube.

It's also great as a time management and scheduling tool alongside a program such as Google Calendar—in fact, I use it to plan out my year monthly, and only then do we as a company go to Google Calendar. My company and many of the other companies, organizations, and schools I have trained use the Switch On Your Brain 5-Step Learning Process for brainstorming, solution-finding and problem-solving, proposal development, streamlining operations, training, strategic and project management, and organizational skills. However, the sky is your limit because the system is training you to think properly and deeply and to build useful and meaningful long-term memory that will forever launch you into success mode.

For the details of how memory forms and the latest on the science of memory and my research, go to chapters 21 and 22. I love these chapters! In fact, I love this whole book, and I hope the techniques and information in this book will help you as much as they have helped me, my family, and hundreds of thousands globally!

Summary of the Switch On Your Brain 5-Step Learning Process

The Switch On Your Brain 5-Step Learning Process builds memory effectively and in an integrated way; builds memory into the dendrites in the brain to ensure information is retained in memory; and ensures that consolidation, integration, and application of knowledge occur. Each step is meticulously designed to stimulate quantum, chemical, and electrical flow through the brain in the most efficient way possible to guarantee meaningful and successful learning. The "thinking-to-understanding" mind-in-action process stimulated by this process will forever change the way you learn and will stretch your potential to untold horizons.

As an *elementary to high school learner*, the five steps will help you think and study correctly.

As a *college learner*, the five steps will help you understand and remember all the information you need to do well on exams, as well as manage the large volumes of work.

As a *teacher*, the five steps will help you transfer the required knowledge to your students 100 percent more effectively. It will also help you teach your students how to think and learn.

As a *trainer*, the five steps will help you decode the material you have to communicate, as well as providing an effective and proven way of transferring the information to your learners.

As a *corporate professional*, the five steps will enhance your knowledge-management ability, improve your reading, help you remember what you have read, help you facilitate meetings, and increase your problem-solving and conflict-management abilities.

In the next section, you will find more intricate details of the timing of memory formation over sixty-three days, including the science of my theory.

SECTION FOUR

The Science

TWENTY-ONE

What Is Memory?

You may have heard or read the popular statement that "nerves that fire together wire together." This phrase refers to the point between neurons where they connect, which is called a synapse (see Image 20.2).

However, we should not take this statement at face value. In this chapter I will be explaining the ins and outs of how memory works within my Geodesic Information Processing Theory. I challenge and add to existing perceptions and theories of memory formation.

Mind in Action

We experience events all the time, all day long. We are also reacting to these events all day long. This is our mind-in-action. This mind-in-action activity is represented in the brain in various ways: quantum, electromagnetic, and electrochemical activity. But not all these events or reactions are remembered later. We can have an experience without actually storing it as a long-term memory. For example, can you remember every detail of how you got to work last Friday, or the details of what your friend told you last month, or even the conversation you had at work yesterday?

We forget certain things because we need to for brain health. We also forget information because we didn't build memory properly, or we build memories incorrectly so we cannot access the information we need. Sometimes we build memories we would rather not remember, which makes us toxic. Our mind and brain health depend on healthy, strong, developing memory. It is toxic to brain tissue if we stop learning; the brain is designed to be grown through deliberate and intentional deep thinking.

Understanding how we think and build memory is how the myth of ADHD can be dispelled and how dementias don't have to become part of the course of life. Many people are misdiagnosed and labeled and put in a box when there wasn't a box to begin with. Instead, everyone should be allowed to develop their customized thinking to build great memory. Everyone can learn how to learn.

The History of Memory

For many years, the prevailing wisdom was that memory was stored in the synaptic connections between neurons. You can pick up any one of those science magazines at the airport with a brain on the cover, and I guarantee it will tell you memory is stored in the intricate net of brain connections between nerve cells. If this truly was the case, we would have a problem. We would not be able to remember much beyond every twenty-four or maybe forty-eight hour period, because this kind of memory formation is short term. Would you go to a doctor who has forgotten what he or she learned twenty-four hours ago? In fact, one of my contracts back in South Africa was to train medical students to build useful long-term memory, to learn how to learn, because, according to the professors who called me in to do this training, "Our medical students can't remember their work." This is definitely not a healthy situation!

Image 21.1

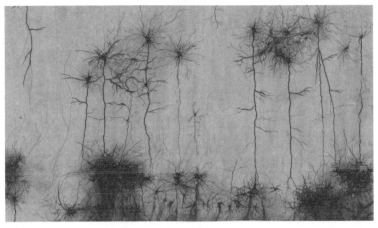

A Golgi stain

So where did we get this mistaken notion of memory formation? This synaptic connection theory was first suggested by Ramon Cajal in 1906 (see Image 21.1).[1] In 1940, Donald Hebb further postulated that nerves that "fire together wire together."[2] This phrase implied that memory is the result of these stronger synaptic connections, which occur when synapses are activated together. At the time, people thought that the tasks of computing—that is, analyzing information to make sense of it (which occurs as signals in the neuron's cell body)—and storing information (which occurs as signals in the dendrites) were one and the same. We now know they are not.[3]

Synaptic connections are, in fact, short-lived. They don't have sufficient storage capacity for the vastness of our memories; they cannot store long-term memories.[4] These synaptic connections are too fluid for long-term memory storage and cannot account for the immense storage capacity of the brain.[5]

Successful Memory

We all want to build the kind of memory that will lead to success. To do so, we need to *think* in such a way that will engage our dendrites to build memory that leads to success in the *long run*. (This is not a quick fix.)

Synaptic connections are a bit like meeting someone for the first time. To get to know them, you have to do more than just meet them once; you need to spend time building a relationship. While synaptic connections represent the initial meeting, building the relationship requires the involvement of the dendrites. Dendrites grow out of the cell body of the neuron (see Image 20.1). Engaging dendrites, like building relationships, is intentional and deliberate and takes a significant investment of your time. The synapses are greatly influenced by the anatomical nonlinear (branched) complexity of the dendrites, with their many ionic voltage gates, which are minute quantum doorways through which ions pass, carrying the information you are learning as electrical and quantum informational messages from the mind.

It is actually very natural to engage dendrites in our thinking, because we naturally think deeply about things that interest us. Things tend to fall apart, however, when we are overwhelmed with too much stimulation, disorganized, impatient, unmotivated, or in toxic stress. These kinds of things can lead to unsuccessful memory formation where information is forgotten or distorted. Of course, this will negatively impact your business meeting, your exam, or even that conversation with your spouse.

You Think Faster Than the Speed of Light

Your thinking is phenomenally fast—every thought you think impacts every single one of the 75 to 100 trillion cells of your body in an instant. Quantum computing in the brain can account for this speed;[6] there are actually certain structures in the brain that facilitate quantum computing and are engaged properly when we think in our customized thinking using the five steps we discussed in section 3.

Quantum means energy: your mind is generating quantum energy through your brain 24/7 as you live, think, and breathe. You need to learn how to make this energy work for you and not against you.

Each thought we think is in fact a veritable universe, as reflected in recent scientific research. Classical physics, which is used to explain voltages and electromagnetic firing of the neurons and synapses, is too slow to account for the speed and infinite nature of our thoughts and the processes we go through as we create them. We thus have to draw on quantum physics to ask the why and how questions of the mind.[7]

Dendrites, working with synapses and cell bodies through quantum action, appear designed to do the job of thinking. As I briefly mentioned, the action of the ions in the little ion voltage gates on the dendrites have quantum qualities.[8] The actual structures that hold the content and attached emotions of our thoughts also operate according to quantum principles.[9] They branch and grow to accommodate the memories of all our manifold, creative experiences, moment by moment of every day, as we learn and build relationships between synapses and dendrites in our brains. This is neuroplasticity in action.

On the other hand, the cell bodies of neurons (see Image 20.2) appear to represent the ongoing experience of thinking in a computational way—that is, the *now* moment of experiencing life in all its diversity.[10]

Quantum Rain Clouds

For just a moment, however, I need to move away from synapses, cell bodies, and dendrites to focus on the clouds of quantum activity that I have briefly mentioned earlier. These quantum effects are actually clouds of probabilities representing all the options and free choices of our minds-in-action.[11] These probabilities are not actual waves but rather waves of probability (possibilities of choices) in a conceptual space that is known as *Hilbert space*.[12] Hilbert space is a mathematical concept named after David Hilbert, one of the most influential mathematicians of the modern era.

The collapse of the wave, or cloud, is the updated knowledge of the observer (you) as you go through the process of thinking, feeling, and choosing in your customized way from the range of probabilities in Hilbert space.[13] These possibilities are, in essence, all the choices that are available to you in any given situation—which can number in the millions! As you analyze (i.e., think and feel), you are in *quantum superposition*. On an atomic level this means two particles are in a 1 and 0 at the same time (which is called a *quibit*) and are being held together by quantum entanglement before they collapse into either a 1 or 0 as the result of a choice—*your* choice. In life, this means you are holding multiple perspectives in view as you compute the potential possibilities of choices that are before you. Should you study for that exam? Should you apologize to that coworker? The possibilities are endless.

The brain, as a quantum computer, can calculate different computations simultaneously in response to the mind-in-action process of decision making. Simply put, we can hold multiple perspectives in mind at the same time. This mind-in-action has physical correlates on multiple levels: from the waves of energy, to the atomic level, and right up to the level of our choosing to believe one reality over another as quantum clouds of probabilities. The power of the mind and brain is breathtaking!

Short-Term Memory

Information (what you are reading, a medical diagnosis, a situation at work, an opportunity, a conversation with a friend, etc.) enters your brain through your five senses and activates electrochemical and quantum action in your neurons and brain. The cell bodies of the neurons are activated in the now moment as you examine the information (as mentioned earlier). At this point in time, the synapses are firing and connections—lots of them!—are forming. As a result, short-term memory is born.[14]

If we go inside the neurons, we find an incredible wonderland: miniscule tubes called *microtubules*, around ten million per neuron.[15] These microtubules are made up of proteins called *tubulin*, which in turn are made up of amino acids called *tryptophan*, which on a molecular level are made up of six carbon atoms in the form of a ring (which is called an *aromatic ring*).[16] Phew! Are you still with me? Hang in there; we will get to the point soon!

Quantum action is taking place at the level of the vibrating electrons oscillating from side to side in this ring. These vibrating electrons, because of Heisenberg's (the founder of quantum physics) *uncertainty principle*,[17] do not have fixed positions (which, on a mind level, means you have not yet made your decision; you are still analyzing, your cells are still computing in response to your mind, and your quantum clouds are still clouding). The electrons therefore spread out like a literal wave or cloud of probabilities (or what you can see as options, possibilities, or tendencies), and the aromatic rings cross over and share electron clouds, going into superpositions of 1 and 0 (the quantum bit or quibit).[18] There is, in fact, not just one pathway of these quibits but several, so they are called *topological quibits*. When they work together it is called *coherence*.[19]

The more we think in our own customized way, the more coherence we will have, enabling us to make positive choices when we are in superposition. As we choose, we select a probability from Hilbert space and collapse the wave (or the cloud).[20] We essentially transform a probability into an actuality or a reality. We turn nothing into a something, which leads to what we say and do.

This collapse of the wave function (or cloud) is also called *decoherence* in quantum theory.[21] As we keep thinking about something, we start building this reality into our brains through genetic expression, allowing the memory building to take place in our dendrites—whatever we think about the most will grow! No wonder quantum physicist Christopher Fuchs calls quantum theory a theory of thought![22]

So, what does all this mean for us? We are constantly building memory and updating our nonconscious mind with new information and increased levels of expertise and wisdom—if we choose correctly. If we choose incorrectly, however, the updated memory knowledge is toxic and brain-damaging. The choice is ours.

The Quantum Zeno Effect

For successful and useful memory to start forming, we need to choose to deliberately and intentionally regulate our thinking through focusing and paying attention to what we allow into our heads. In quantum physics, this means we activate the *Quantum Zeno Effect* (QZE), which is a type of decoherence effect where the clouds of quantum activity collapse (*decohere*) as a result of what we think, feel, and choose, and a physical memory is built.[23]

The QZE describes how, when we repeatedly pay attention to something, which collapses a wave function or cloud of possibilities, we are creating a long-term memory that will become part of our belief systems and influence our choices in the future. In simple terms, the QZE is the repeated *effort* that makes learning take place. Whatever we think about the most will grow.

Short-Term and Long-Term Memory

As we saw above, synaptic connections that occur after the activity in the cell body and after the collapsing of the clouds account for short-term memory, due to their transient nature. The dendrites will eventually store that experience as a long-term memory, provided there is deliberate, intentional thinking and ongoing stimulation over a period of about three weeks, which happens when you use my Switch On You Brain 5-Step Learning Process. A fleeting experience activates cell body activity and connections at the synapse, building short-term memory. Deep, deliberate thinking to understand and remember, on the other hand, activates synaptic connections, cell body activity, and dendritic activity, which leads to useful long-term memory.

Successful long-term memory requires more time and more work. To build useful long-term memories, we have to do something more than just experience something or some piece of information in the now moment. We have to deliberately and intentionally think to understand in order to build memory and, hence, to learn. This kind of successful memory formation has been the objective of my work, and hence this book, and exactly why I have said there are three parts to mental self-care: mindsets, customized thinking, and learning.

When we are going through life—for example, when we are at school listening to a lecture or at work listening to an instruction from a boss—we will experience:

- Quantum clouds of activity in the brain.
- Computational activity in the cell body.
- The synaptic strength increasing as we think about the situation, because this thinking causes repeated firing of synapses—that is, high-frequency stimulation at the synapses. This is called long-term potentiation (LTP), which, in older theories of memory, was erroneously seen as long-term memory. In reality, this firing is short-term memory, as we discussed above, which has the *potential* to become long-term memory.
- The deeper and more deliberate our thinking is, the more we will activate the dendrites to grow, which allows long-term memory to start forming.

The more you practice deliberate, self-regulatory thinking by using the techniques in this book, the more your brain will respond—you are literally redesigning your brain as you think! The dendrites will actually start to grow bumps, called spines, that look a bit like the nodes on a branch when a new branch forms on a tree (see Image 20.1).[24] These bumps change shape over time in response to *daily*, *deep*, *deliberate* thinking.

The bump, however, is a weak memory. As it becomes a lollipop shape it is getting stronger; once it looks like a mushroom these memories are the strongest and most self-sustainable. Essentially, the spines on the dendrites indicate long-term memory as more and more lump-shaped spines transform into long-term memory mushroom-shaped spines.

The converse also applies. The synapses need constant activity to maintain their strength, so when you do not think as deeply or regularly about something, or if you stop thinking about it completely, the activity relating to this will be reduced or stop, and the synapse will lose energy and therefore strength. As a result, the proteins around the sensitive synapse will disappear, and there is a decrease in dendritic spines and dendrites; the proteins denature (die off) and we forget about the thing or experience. This process of forgetting is called long-term depression or LTD.[25]

It is incredibly important to remember that whether this information gets stored in the dendrites or not depends on how *intentionally* we think about something, and how much time and effort is expended thinking about this thing. What we remember and learn is in our hands.

Three Levels of Thinking

In effect, there are three levels of thinking. This relates back to the Switch On Your Brain 5-Step Learning Process, discussed in the previous chapter. In fact, let me remind you that this chapter relates to this process and to the entire book as the underlying scientific principles. So, when you apply the techniques of the previous chapters, you are doing all the great things described in this section!

Level one contains thoughts that are just fleeting, which will disappear very quickly, within twenty-four to forty-eight hours, if not sooner.[26] No deep thinking is involved, and no dendrites or extra dendritic spines are formed. Only the cell body, synaptic connections, and quantum clouds are activated. Level two involves more deliberate thinking. However, if after a few days you stop feeding the memory, you will forget most of it. Dendrites and spines grow, but as they were not stabilized and automatized, most decrease and disappear in a short period of time. This will occur if you stop working on something between five to fourteen *consecutive* days. The third level of thinking involves constant, deliberate, and intentional activity daily for at least three consecutive weeks. This type of thinking builds strong dendrites with mushroom spines, which are long-term memories. The Switch On Your Brain 5-Step Learning Process effectively activates all these levels.

A memory is only useful if you automatize it. *Automatization* is the science of habit building. This simply means the memory is turned into a habit through a process that takes more than twenty-one days.

In order for a memory to be usable, it needs lots of energy. It gets lots of "packets" of energy (*quanta*) when you repeatedly think about the memory daily, through the disciplined process of going through all five steps of my program, which results in the required neurochemical and structural changes in the brain that make this memory a usable and useful thought. This is the QZE I discussed above; repeated effort makes learning take place. Intentional daily focus over a minimum of sixty-three days, in twenty-one-day cycles, allows a habit to form.[27]

A useful memory, therefore, has lots of energy, making it an *accessible* memory. When a memory becomes accessible, it informs the next decision, such as informing the answer on an exam. If you do not automatize the memory, however, it will not be accessible and therefore not helpful to you. In order to turn long-term memory into habits, you will have to choose the hard work route of investing time, specifically sixty-three days, in repeatedly thinking about new information. You saw how to apply this when you worked through the Switch On Your Brain 5-Step Learning Process in chapter 20.

Unfortunately, most people give up within the first week of learning and do not push through. As a result, they have to start learning all over again, which is not only tedious and disheartening but also creates negative feedback loops. Quick fixes and memory tricks are illusions—do not let them fool you.

Customized Thinking Gets Memories Building

Your customized mode of thinking gets activity going on a quantum level and electromagnetically in the cell body of the neuron, which is where information is computed and transmitted. This is your mind-in-action, which has a causal effect in your physical brain. The deeper and more intentionally you think to understand, remember, and apply this information, the more you will cycle through your seven stages of thought in your gift, and the more you will move beyond computation, transmission, and connecting synapses to actively engaging the dendrites, where information is stored as a long-term memory.[28]

The deep thinking induced by my Switch On Your Brain 5-Step Learning Process uses your customized way of thinking and allows for the signals between dendrites, cell bodies, and synapses of the neurons to be highly synchronized, which is important for effective memory building for both learning new information and detoxing mind issues. This process allows useful and meaningful memories to develop, which can help you succeed in every area of your life. Indeed, you cannot be successful in school, work, and life if you can't remember or don't have understanding of the relevant and pertinent information for that situation.

Very often we go into situations with desynchronized information, recognizing we know about something but unable to remember enough to contribute or be effective and successful in the moment. By using the Gift Profile and Switch On Your Brain

5-Step Learning Process, you can learn how to use your mind to your advantage and avoid this kind of situation.

But What about the Dendrites?

I have talked a lot about building memory into the dendrites, but what actually happens inside the dendrites when long-term memory is stored? Dendrites not only increase in number, strength, and length as you deliberately think about something but, as briefly mentioned above, also have spines on them, which are a bit like the nodes on tree branches where other branches grow from. Thinking deeply and deliberately makes them grow and become denser, and the spines change into a mushroom shape. The way dendritic spine density changes has a lot to do with memory.

The changes in the dendrites *appear* to mainly occur in the prefrontal cortex and hippocampus. However, as science advances, we may see more areas of the brain implicated. Yet, at this stage in memory research, we believe that short-term memory generally happens in the hippocampus, long-term memory appears to be stored in dendrites in the neocortex, and perceptual memory is in the amygdala.[29]

As discussed earlier, a pattern emerges where the formation of a memory starts with thinking about something; this leads to quantum action and an initial electrical alteration in the cell bodies and synapses of cells potentially in the hippocampus, which initiates a series of structural changes that lead to strengthening of synaptic function and long-term potentiation (LTP). Over time this initial change is translated into further, more persistent structural changes in the dendrites and dendritic spines.

It is important to note that despite centuries of research, encoding in the brain has remained quite mysterious. Memories last a lifetime; however, synaptic connections are short-lived, suggesting memory is stored at a deeper level. It appears that microtubules, which are the major components of the structural cytoskeleton within neurons as I discussed above, provide this mechanism.[30]

Microtubules in dendrites are broken up into branches and therefore are ideal for memory storage. Microtubules are made of the protein tubulin (mentioned earlier), which forms 15 percent of total brain protein. Microtubules regulate synapses, define the architecture of neurons, and appear to process information through their tubulin components, which act like mini quantum computers.[31]

Snowflakes and Walking Nano Poodles

Wait, what? Snowflakes? Mushrooms? Nano Poodles? Bear with me! I understand that the description of memory formation can be complicated, but, if nothing else, this section highlights the power and complexity of our minds and brains. It is a reminder of how powerful our thinking really is!

As we think, the mind-in-action signal causes activity at the pre-synapse, which, in turn, activates prolonged activity on the other side of the synapse (see Image 20.2). This pre-synaptic activation involves calcium ions, which carry the electromagnetic and quantum form of the information. Imagine a shopping bag holding your clothes. They pass into the post-synaptic neurons through little doorways called *receptors*. Once inside, they activate Camk11, which is an essential protein player in memory that looks like a snowflake. These "snowflakes" are subsequently transformed into a six-legged shape that is fondly called a Nano Poodle.[32] It's as though the shopping bag contains a new outfit, and when you put it on you are transformed and ready for that party.

Extensive research by Sir Roger Penrose and Professor Stuart Hamerhoff has shown that the Nano Poodles land on the tubulin. Each leg of a Nano Poodle (called a *kinase domain*) is able to deposit information in the form of energy via *phosphorylation* (the mechanism by which the activity of proteins is altered after they are formed; a phosphate group is added to a protein by specific enzymes called *kinases*).[33] This encodes one bit of synaptic information for a long time and then moves on; it is a memory trace.

Extensive research by Sir Roger Penrose and Professor Stuart Hamerhoff has shown that the Nano Poodles deposit information into the tubulin because they perfectly match the spatial dimensions, geometry, and electrostatic binding of tubulin, like a puzzle piece. The tubulin is therefore known as the intra-neuronal substrate for memory, the minute quantum computer encoding the actual place where your thoughts are physically stored.[34]

Centrioles, which are made up of these tubulin microtubules, are involved in cell division, which is a language of sorts. The centrioles store epigenetic memory; here, behaviors are transferred generationally and affect how we function physically.[35] This is an excellent example of the mind-body connection.

The brain is richly populated with these microtubules and Nano Poodles. These structures are capable of information processing at the level of the membranes and cytoskeletal elements of a cell.[36]

Wrinkles and Rust

Tubulins have another really interesting characteristic: they self-assemble and reassemble. They are entropy-driven, which is highly unusual because the second law of thermodynamics basically states that entropy always increases with time—rust and wrinkles are good examples of this! Tubulins essentially go against this law, a significant feat that allows neurons to grow and therefore memories to develop.[37]

It takes thousands to tens of thousands of tubulins to make one microtubule, and in one neuron there are billions of tubulins that make up all the microtubules. Each tubulin has water around it, and they are attached in an ordered way. When they assemble, they lose most of the water, so the net gain in disorder is greater than the net gain in order. This means the microtubule assembly is more disorderly than the individual tubulins floating around. This is important because it actually provides insight into the physical correlate for randomness—the randomness of free will.[38] This disorderliness reflects the infinite and ever-changing nature of our thoughts. We need a structure that can handle our choices, and tubulin and quantum clouds seem well suited to do the job.

In all cells, microtubules are arranged continuously from the center of the cell outward like spokes of a wheel. This is the *cyto-skeletal structure*. Neurons have the most microtubules because they are the most complicated in terms of their structure. In dendrites, however, the microtubules are short, interrupted, and in mixed polarity networks, so they are not providing skeletal support. Rather, they have some other function. According to anesthetist and consciousness researcher Stuart Hameroff, this structure is perfect for providing information processing and memory storage.[39]

Hameroff believes that tubulin gives us a glimpse into the mind-blowing power of the mind, pun intended! Each neuron has approximately 10^9 (one billion) tubulins, which are the subunits of the microtubule. Tubulins are the equivalent of a bit because they are changing every second; in fact, they switch about a million times a second in the megahertz range. This means you have about 10^{16} operations per second *in a single neuron*.[40]

Artificial intelligence researchers believe that once computation gets complex enough, which they assume is 10^{16}, then artificial beings will produce intelligent consciousness and develop the same wisdom and understanding as humans do. However, according to Hameroff, they are going on the assumption that 10^{16} is the total ops per second for the whole brain, yet it is actually only for one neuron—and there are about 100 billion neurons in the brain. As Hameroff shows, if you therefore multiply 10^{16} by 100 billion neurons, the power in the brain is actually about 10^{27} (approximately 400 billion) operations per second![41]

As Hameroff also notes, we need to look deeper inside the neurons to the microtubules and the tubulin, which act as incredible quantum computers. These structures connect with the universe at the quantum level, processing information and generating energy at these incomprehensible speeds. According to Penrose and Hamer-hoff, they potentially go ever deeper into levels of space-time geometry, a possibility that is consistent with many notions of human spirituality. There is a lot more going on in the mind than we realize, which we are starting to see through research in quantum physics and quantum biology. This is an exciting time to be alive!

The Quantum Angle of the Geodesic Model

The brain responds to the mind. Quantum theory is a way of understanding this interaction between the mind and the brain; it uses mathematics to describe this relationship.[42]

Indeed, the human brain, as the substrate through which the mind works, cannot be explained by classical physics alone. The more we examine and understand human consciousness and the power of choice, the more we see that humans are not just complicated biological machines of cause and effect. As quantum physicist Henry Stapp asks,

> How do the motions of the miniature planet-like objects of classical physics give rise to individualistic feelings and understanding and knowing? Classical physics says one day these connections will be known, but how can they be understood in terms of a theory . . . that eliminates the agent of the "connection"[?][43]

Classical physics cannot describe our unique experiences. Rather, it operates in a predetermined physical world concerned with actualities rather than the potentialities of the human mind. In quantum physics, however, we can see how we are players in a game; we are cocreators of our evolving physical reality.

The Individual Observer

Werner Heisenberg, who received the Nobel Prize in 1932 for the creation of quantum physics, proposed a quantum generalization of classical laws. Heisenberg's replacement of numbers by actions incorporated the individual observer into the core of quantum mechanics. The number represents "internal properties of a physical system," whereas the action that replaces the number represents the person with their free will observing or probing the system. Actions replacing numbers challenges the materialism of classical physics, for the mind (the individual observer) freely changes the brain (the physical realm). In essence, the freely chosen, conscious intentions and perceptions of the individual are injected into a physical system (brain), changing it structurally. This, in turn, results in words and actions, and more physical change occurs in our brains and thus in our world.

Heisenberg could not, however, explain what causes changes in the brain.[44] Laws cannot generate by themselves; they need someone or something to generate them. John von Neumann's form of quantum mechanics solved this problem by introducing the individual with his or her free choices, which filled Heisenberg's causal gap.[45]

The mind-brain quantum theory is called the Von Neumann Orthodox Formulation of Quantum Mechanics (a mouthful, I know!).[46] It is built around the effect of a person's psychologically described and intentional actions on physically described properties (i.e., the person's brain). It specifies the causal connections between the realm of the mind and the realm of the brain, which are governed by the basic laws of physics. This formulation overcomes the main objection to Cartesian dualism, which is the lack of an understanding of how the mind can affect the brain. Notably, it shows that human consciousness cannot be "an inert witness to the mindless dance of atoms."[47] We have a lot of control over what goes on inside our heads. We are not merely dancing to the tune of our atoms or our DNA.

As we saw above, the brain has a quantum nature, shown by quantum physics calculations and quantum neurobiology, that cannot be adequately explained by classical physics. For example, ionic processes occurring in nerves, which are at the atomic level and cannot be accounted for by classical physics alone because they are too small, control the brain. The process of exocytosis, for example, which deals with the dumping of neurotransmitter molecules into the synapses, requires the more fine-tuned explanations of quantum mechanics.[48]

Quantum theory evinces the importance of the mind-in-action, the mind-brain connection, and the power of our intellect, will, and emotions, which can cause physical changes in the brain. As a result, quantum theory is a very powerful way of explaining learning and memory, alongside neuroscience and neuropsychology. For this reason, I have incorporated it into the development of my theory, The Geodesic Information Processing Theory (see next chapter) to explain the mind-brain connection.

Philosopher and theologian Keith Ward calls quantum theory "the most accurate model ever developed to understand the deepest things."[49] Two of the "deepest things," two of the biggest questions we all face at one time or another, are how we uniquely think as human beings and what our purpose on this earth is. Why do we have the minds we do? Quantum physics gives us a way of describing, scientifically, this innate sense of purpose by showing us how powerful our minds are. It provides a scientific theory that explains the power of an individual's ability to choose, and thus to change his or her brain, body, and the world. It highlights the importance of thinking and how we are all unique. Quantum physics thus provides validation of something we all sense intuitively: our conscious thoughts have the power to affect our actions.

Entanglement

Quantum physics helps us understand just how entangled and dependent our world is. If a photon comes into existence a billion light-years from here, it affects you, even if you do not notice it affecting you. John Bell, famous for Bell's Theorem (formulated at CERN in Geneva in 1964),[50] observed that there is an inseparable quantum connectedness of every part with every other part in our universe. No matter how far apart in distance and time, all particles in a relationship affect each other; these relationships exist beyond space and time.

TWENTY-TWO

The Geodesic Information Processing Theory

You have made it to the last chapter, well done! In this chapter, you will learn about the scientific research underpinning everything you have read about in this book. You don't have to read it to benefit from the book, but I have chosen to include this heavy science section, written as simply as I can, to help you understand the foundation of my principles. Of course, these are complex concepts. Yet they are very relevant to understanding the point of mental self-care and going beyond mindfulness.

The Geodesic Information Processing Theory is the theory that I first developed nearly thirty years ago and have updated in the intervening years. The tools presented in this book are based on this foundation, as are all my programs and books.[1] The Gift Profile and the Switch On Your Brain 5-Step Learning Process were developed out of this model.

As you read through this section, it will be helpful to refer back to Image 22.1, the model of my theory.

My theory has several different components:

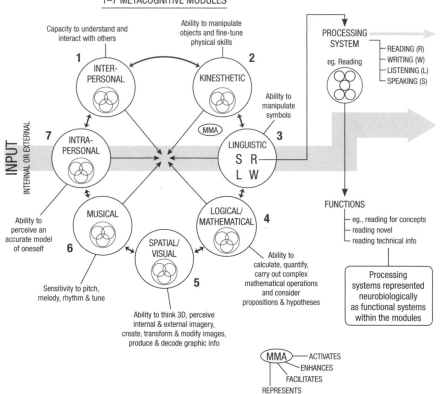

Image 22.1

THE GEODESIC INFORMATION PROCESSING MODEL

NONCONSCIOUS

METACOGNITIVE LEVEL

90% of Learning

MMA

| Root of thinking process and then structure of the non-conscious | → | Automatized complex higher cortical functions |

1–7 METACOGNITIVE MODULES

Capacity to understand and interact with others

Ability to manipulate objects and fine-tune physical skills

PROCESSING SYSTEM

eg. Reading

— READING (R)
— WRITING (W)
— LISTENING (L)
— SPEAKING (S)

1 INTER-PERSONAL

2 KINESTHETIC

Ability to manipulate symbols

7 INTRA-PERSONAL

MMA

3 LINGUISTIC

S R
L W

INPUT
INTERNAL OR EXTERNAL

MUSICAL

LOGICAL/ MATHEMATICAL **4**

FUNCTIONS

— eg., reading for concepts
— reading novel
— reading technical info

6
Ability to perceive an accurate model of oneself

SPATIAL/ VISUAL

5

Ability to calculate, quantify, carry out complex mathematical operations and consider propositions & hypotheses

Sensitivity to pitch, melody, rhythm & tune

Ability to think 3D, perceive internal & external imagery, create, transform & modify images, produce & decode graphic info

| Processing systems represented neurobiologically as functional systems within the modules |

MMA ——ACTIVATES
——ENHANCES
——FACILITATES
REPRESENTS

NEUROPSYCHOLOGICAL LEVEL

| BIOLOGICAL REPRESENTATION |

| 1–7 represented biologically as modular columns of neuronal cells ascending from the cortex to the subcortex to the limbic system across the left and right hemispheres |

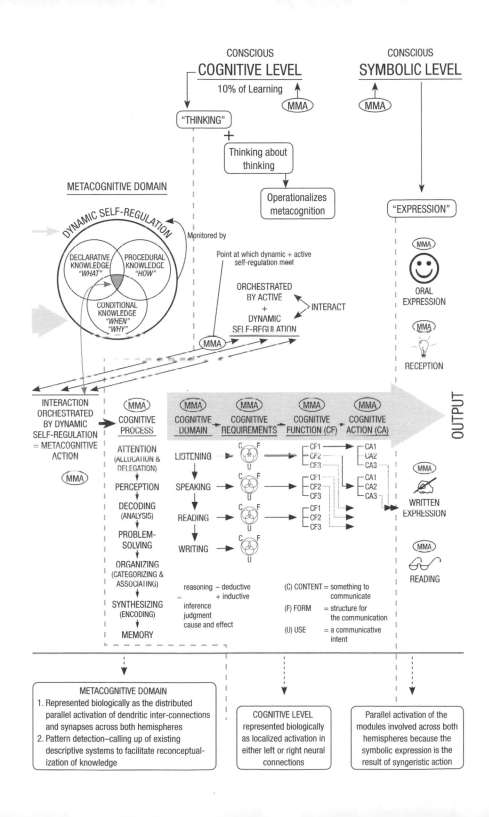

- There are *seven metacognitive modules*: Interpersonal, Intrapersonal, Linguistic, Logical/Mathematical, Kinesthetic, Musical, and Visual/Spatial.
- Each metacognitive module has four *processing systems*: Speaking, Reading, Writing, and Listening.
- Each processing system is broken down into three *metacognitive domains*: the Declarative (the "what" of the information of the memory), the Procedural (the "how" of the information of the memory), and the Conditional (the "when/why," or the purpose and emotional component of the memory).
- These metacognitive domains provide the structure of the *descriptive systems* (memories). The exclusivity of your memories is housed within these three elements.
- The activity happening in these components is controlled by mind-in-action regulation—your thinking, feeling, and choosing. On a nonconscious level, where approximately 90 to 99 percent of learning takes place, this is called *dynamic self-regulation*. On a conscious level, where only approximately 1 to 10 percent of learning takes place, this is called *active self-regulation*.
- Finally, *metacognitive action* is the term for the deep thinking that causes the what, how, and when/why elements of your memory to start interacting through deliberate, intentional thinking. The more intentional and deliberate the active self-regulation, the more likely it is to interact with dynamic self-regulation (nonconscious level).
- The *memories with the most energy*—the memories, which are thoughts, that have had repeated, effortful attention paid to them and are therefore embedded in an accessible format—will move into the conscious mind. Whatever moves into conscious awareness is thus what we have spent the most time thinking about.

The Seven Metacognitive Modules

All seven metacognitive modules work together in an entangled fashion. More specifically, these modules work in unique ways for each of us. The seven metacognitive modules of the gift structure/ design are housed within the complex, quantum nonconscious mind, which works 24/7 at vast speeds estimated at 10^{27}.

These seven modules are not exhaustive but rather representative of the broad range of human knowledge and intellectual potential. All individuals possess the full spectrum of all seven metacognitive modules, but in varying amounts and combined in different ways, thus revealing specific cognitive features—hence the specificity of your customized mode of thinking, as identified in the Gift Profile we studied in section 2.

The seven metacognitive modules of my theory differ from the seven intelligences of Howard Gardner's "multiple intelligences" theory.[2] My seven modules incorporate all three types of knowledge within the metacognitive domain: declarative, procedural, and conditional knowledge. Gardner's intelligences only incorporate procedural knowledge and are therefore incomplete in the sense of the range of human knowledge.

We cannot approach the way we think, feel, and choose in a reductionist manner. Even though these modules function as independent units, each with their own cognitive characteristics, they are designed to interact as you process information (thinking, feeling, and choosing). When these modules interact, higher-order thinking is produced, because the net result of interaction between the modules is improved quality *within* the modules.

It is important to remember that the seven metacognitive modules work in harmony. You can't observe or listen to a person and notice all seven. What you will see is the end product of all seven modules working together in a way that is unique to that person. It is the collective whole that is expressed through someone's words and actions that gives each of us our own "harmony."

231

The Processing Systems

As I mentioned above, the metacognitive modules are divided into four processing systems: read, speak, listen, and write. Each of these processing systems in turn has a function, such as reading for concepts, reading a novel for pleasure, reading a complex technical manual, writing an email, writing a story, giving a speech, having a conversation with your best friend, and so on.

A processing system is a result of a whole arrangement of processes. For example, the processing system of reading a book, which would be part of the Linguistic metacognitive module, is made up of various processes such as the visual tracking of letters, the visual discrimination of letters, and the combining of these letters into units of meaning. The processing system of reading also has various functions, such as reading for factual knowledge or reading to learn what happens to characters in a novel. We each have our own interpretation/filter (our customized mode of thinking) as we are doing this.

A processing system is represented neurologically as a functional structure composed of interrelations of different parts of the brain. Processing systems will eventually be expressed on the symbolic level by cognitive action—what you say and what you do (see Image 22.1). On my model, a processing system is viewed as the channel through which the intellectual abilities specific to a particular domain are expressed.

Functioning in your customized thinking and using the Switch On Your Brain 5-Step Learning Process will maximize the selection and integration of functions into the most efficient processing systems to operationalize the cognitive acts, resulting in optimal performance. This means you will say and do the best for that situation.

Dynamic Self-Regulation

In order to be able to read that book or give that speech, you need to activate or operationalize the processing system. This is called *dynamic self-regulation,* a very powerful driving force of your nonconscious mind-in-action and one very specific to your customized thinking.

As mentioned above, your nonconscious mind is always in action 24/7, so dynamic self-regulation is always going on. Your nonconscious mind does not stop analyzing, cleaning up, reading, and integrating all the memories you have, which are changing and growing in response to the experiences of your daily life.

Ultimately, the activity of the nonconscious mind accounts for the high-level decision-making action that is going on even when we get distracted with other tasks on a conscious level. Dynamic self-regulation controls up to 90 percent of thinking and learning. It is responsible for activating and energizing long-term memories and belief systems (worldviews) to move into our conscious awareness and, as such, has an enormous influence on our conscious thinking, feeling, and choosing. Dynamic self-regulation also maintains awareness and alertness in the seven metacognitive modules as internal reconstruction (redesigning, growing, and changing of memories) is taking place.

Active Self-Regulation

Conscious, cognitive thinking is called *active self-regulation.* The deeper we think, the more active self-regulation interacts with dynamic self-regulation. Active self-regulation is intentional and controlled by your choice to pay attention to something. Its effectiveness is determined by how mindful and deliberate you are in any given moment.

It is important to remember that thoughts (also known as descriptive systems or memories) are automatized (made into a habit) through deliberate, repeated, and conscious cognitive thinking. This type of thinking has to occur for a minimum of three cycles of twenty-one days (so sixty-three days) in order for true understanding to take place.

The Metacognitive Domain and Descriptive Systems

Each of the seven metacognitive modules uses its own operating system, known as the *metacognitive domain*. These domains use declarative (what), procedural (how), and conditional (when/why) types of knowledge to build pattern-nature memories (descriptive systems). These memories, in turn, grow into belief systems or worldviews, which are reflected in our attitudes (expanded and strengthened descriptive systems).

Every moment of every day we are merging with our environment. Through thinking, feeling, and choosing, we are learning and planting thoughts, which are real, physical things, into the brain. This sophisticated and complex process is essentially the expansion and solidification of descriptive systems through the addition of the three types of knowledge (thinking, feeling, and choosing) to the metacognitive domain. It happens in our minds 24/7, even when we are asleep! We truly are superbly intellectual beings, even when we are not aware of what is going on in our minds.

Yet what occurs on the metacognitive level is unique for each of us. The particular way you build and store memories is based on your specific perceptions and interpretations, which are exclusive to you. The various mechanisms in the nervous system are, in fact, activated to carry out specific operations on the information, and structural change occurs in the brain—and this is unique for each person. The repeated use of, elaboration of, and interaction among the computational devices will lead to forms of knowledge that are useful, intelligent, and exclusive to you. Thus, the metacognitive domains in the geodesic model reflect the idea that human beings are so constituted as to be sensitive to certain information in their own unique way.

When a particular form of information is presented, your mind goes into action and works through the substrate of your brain. Your self-regulation will be completely different from mine; the person thinking in his or her default mode of thinking drives all these processes.

In the Geodesic Information Processing Theory, memory is essentially seen as part of the cognitive process, where the new descriptive systems are reconceptualized or redesigned. Once a new descriptive system is reconceptualized, it is stored in the appropriate metacognitive domains of the specified metacognitive modules in the form of declarative, procedural, and conditional knowledge. The reconceptualization of new knowledge is actualized and enhanced on the cognitive level, then stored on the metacognitive level, where it will be used in the future reconceptualization of new knowledge.

Metacognitive Action and Readiness Potential

Mindful, intentional, and deliberate active self-regulation will activate interaction between active and dynamic self-regulation, the result of which is thinking deeply. This deep thinking is called *metacognitive action*, which is when the what, how, and when/why elements of your memory start interacting through deliberate thinking until they generate enough energy to move into your conscious mind. If conscious thinking is not deliberate (that is, with the aim to develop understanding, which is when active and dynamic self-regulation interact), over a period of approximately sixty-three days, then what you are thinking about will not become an influential part of your nonconscious mind.[3] These are the processes you have been learning to activate in this book.

Intentional, deep thinking shapes our worldview. These thoughts become deeply rooted in the nonconscious mind and, even though they are not available to conscious introspection, they still influence the cognitive end-products of our thinking, feeling, and choosing. They become available to conscious introspection only when we think deeply, using our customized mode of thinking, which literally gives them the energy to move into conscious awareness.

Metacognitive action is your deep thinking, feeling, and choosing, expressed as the fundamental elements of the way you think. As the memory bubbles up into the conscious part of your mind, you become aware of it, and the memory influences or doesn't influence—you can consciously choose—your current processing of whatever it is you are focusing on. And, as the relevant memories move from the nonconscious to the conscious mind, experience is enlarged and increased with new knowledge added to the memories. Better integration among memories will occur the deeper we think, also contributing to the reconceptualization of knowledge. Essentially, we don't just add facts to our memories; we literally redesign them with each new piece of information we uniquely perceive and understand. If a person is not deeply thinking—thinking, feeling, and choosing in a repeated, intentional, deliberate way and taking responsibility for his or her learning—the input will not be strong enough to induce cognitive, emotional, behavioral, and academic change.

As mentioned throughout this book, when we think deeply in our unique way (see chapter 18 on the Gift Profile) and use the Switch On Your Brain 5-Step Learning Process, we induce neuroplasticity: our brains change. Our minds read or interpret the activities and patterns of the neurons and dendrites of our brains. Dendrites store the memories made by the signals of the mind (see chapter 20). The more we think and generate metacognitive action, the more we influence and change this configuration of the physical memory, which is then ready to be read again (remembered) at a later time through metacognitive action. This all requires the brain to function properly.

Scientists see traces of this nonconscious dynamic self-regulation activity in the brain, which is called the *readiness potential*. This potential involves the interaction between dynamic and active self-regulation that is activated through deliberate, deep thinking. Once this interaction occurs, the cognitive process is literally switched on. Cognition is regulated by metacognition and carries the metacognitive action of the processing system through to the symbolic expressive level—what we say and do. And as you use the techniques in this book, you are activating these processes.

The Question of Consciousness

Benjamin Libet, a pioneer in the field of human consciousness, performed one of the first studies on cognition and metacognition.[4] His research began in the early 1980s (when I was doing my first level of graduate research in this field) and has shaped the way many scientists approach the question of consciousness. Libet connected people to a machine that measured brain activity while they were asked to randomly decide to press a button. The subjects were then asked to consciously note when they decided to press the button. He found that just prior to the conscious decision to press the button—approximately 200 milliseconds—there was a conscious buildup of activity in the brain, which he coined the "readiness potential." At approximately 350 milliseconds the subjects showed unconscious activity before reporting any degree of conscious awareness. Later studies saw this buildup ten seconds prior to a conscious decision.[5]

Some adherents of materialism interpreted Libet's findings in a way that negated the power of choice. They concluded that the studies showed that the brain was the cause of conscious activity, since the buildup of readiness potential occurred prior to a conscious decision.[6] Subsequently, they used this interpretation to deny the existence of free will. More research showed, however, that the readiness potential was still there even when subjects had to push a button when they saw a cube among many other shapes.[7] Measured brain activity during the task showed that the readiness potential was there even before the stimuli appeared. As one of the researchers noted,

Our results show that neural activity, which is present prior to motor responses, emerges well before the presentation of a stimulus. At that time the participants were not capable of knowing whether to press the left- or right-hand button before a stimulus appeared. In addition, the activation preceding the stimulation did not differ significantly between the two response alternatives. Thus, the observed activity cannot be regarded as a specific preparation to press one of the buttons rather than the other one.[8]

In essence, we cannot say that the "brain decided" to press one button. Readiness potential exists whether or not there is a button to press (or some other stimulus); something else is responsible for the specific decisions we make at any given moment. We cannot look at a brain and decide why a human being makes the choices he or she makes, because the brain with its neural correlates does not tell us about a person's experience and free will.

Libet, in fact, did not deny free will.[9] He noted that the mind had the ability to veto an action while neural activity continued. He called this the "conscious veto," which supports the idea of free will. The brain will run on autopilot and carry out tasks, yet the unique and complex mind or "self" (customized thinking) has the ability to interfere by preventing activity from being carried out.

These studies do not merely demonstrate that the brain runs on autopilot. Free will is not just an illusion, as several prominent materialists would have us believe.[10] Rather, the brain, as a physical substrate, appears to be responding to (or is being "used" by) the nonconscious mind, which is orchestrated by dynamic self-regulation and the process of selecting the appropriate descriptive systems (memories) that need to move to the conscious mind. Once the memories have moved into the conscious mind and we filter the information through our customized mode of thinking, we think, feel, and make a choice about whether to comply with or override an action. What we choose matters.

The Difference between Your Customized Thinking and Mine

The difference between your customized thinking and mine appears to involve differences in the components of the seven metacognitive modules, their metacognitive domains, and their processing systems. Indeed, the metacognitive action of both dynamic and active self-regulation is also exclusive to the individual. How you drive your mind is unique: your customized way of thinking is captured and reflected in the what, how, and when/why, plus how you manage these through dynamic and active self-regulation.

As you worked through the Gift Profile, this exclusivity of your customized thinking is what you were unlocking. The net result is a mindful awareness of your identity: it is a particular insight into your customized thinking so you can enhance and improve your ability to think, feel, and choose. This is intelligent mindfulness. All seven metacognitive modules work together in a simultaneous, entangled fashion, and in unique ways for each of us. We all have the ability to think, feel, and choose, but our customized thinking is different and exclusively our own, just like our fingerprints. Strength in the sum of the parts is the fundamental principle of this modular perspective. The quality of higher cortical functions is influenced by the harmonious interaction of the seven metacognitive modules.

When we move out of our customized thinking, we do not tap into the modules correctly. Incorrect thinking only taps into a selection of modules, and does so in a partial manner. We should therefore be very aware of what we are focusing on: we could be learning things that will have a negative impact on our health. Using the techniques presented in this book will enable you to think yourself into success mode.

Learning

Learning is the creative reconceptualization of knowledge. It is the redesigning of memory. It is controlled by active and dynamic self-regulation. It has the quality of personal involvement, it is pervasive, and its essence is meaning and purpose. What we learn determines the meaning of our lives, since it shapes our worldview—or the mindset filter through which we see everything.

When we operate in our customized thinking and use the Switch On Your Brain 5-Step Learning Process, we are learning in a healthy way and building healthy memories. New developments in the field of experimental physics confirm the need for this type of deep, focused-learning approach to memory formation, which I have used successfully for over three decades in my work and research.[11] However, when we operate outside of this, we learn in a distorted way and build toxic memories that damage the brain and body. We all have to ask ourselves what we want in the memory storages of our minds. Whatever we focus on the most will grow and influence our perspectives and belief systems (or worldviews). As the saying goes, we become what we love. This can be both a positive and negative experience.

Operating in your customized thinking, incorporating the correct mindsets, and applying the Switch On Your Brain 5-Step Learning Process will make a world of difference to your thinking, learning, and succeeding.

Epilogue

M indsets contain power; customized thinking activates this power; the five-step process builds this power into long-term, sustainable change.

Mindsets are the frame; they are also the canvas and the paints. Customized thinking is the power of the process of painting, a process that will be different for each of us. Memory building is the finished artwork hanging in our gallery. And you—you are the genius, painting a masterpiece no one has ever painted before.

You cannot control the events and circumstances of life. You can, however, control your reactions to the events and circumstances of life through the choices you make and the thoughts you think. When you understand the power of your mindsets and your customized way of thinking and harness the power in your mind to build healthy memories, you will begin to realize that you can choose to control how you live your life. You can choose what painting you want to create!

The tools in this book are designed to help you thrive and not just survive. They will help you learn to harness the power of your thoughts to think deeply, learn powerfully, deal with the perils of our digital age, and live a life filled with meaning.

You are able to discover success as you think and learn at school, at work, and in every area of your life. You are not a victim of what people say about you or what you say about yourself. Regardless of where you are and what happens to you, you can live the kind of life you want to live.

The choice is *yours*.

Afterword

With our ever-increasing awareness of the intricate connectedness of all of the macrocosm "outside" of us, and the ever-expanding microcosm "inside" of us, this new text by Dr. Leaf should become a required read-and-study for every adult. It is a call to awareness of the cataclysmic decline in true learning arising from our societal trend away from true thinking skills and leading to a destructive and empty definition of what society defines as success.

Dr. Leaf again brings to the forefront how our thinking—our mindset—essentially guides the efficacy of our learning. As she states in her introduction, "We are not designed to remember everything and anything. We are designed to remember what we need to succeed. This requires comprehension and deep, focused understanding. We need to learn what to learn and how to learn."

With most humans increasingly being bombarded with information from our youngest ages, more and more are experiencing "incessant chatter" that is ceaselessly hijacking our minds, our thoughts, our emotions, and our actions. We have been witnessing and experiencing a global shift in the "way" we are thinking, and the results are not good—whether one analyzes the data from the CDC, the NIMH, the WHO, or any other organization accurately tracking the epidemic decrease in our overall mental health—including an epidemic increase in neurophysiologically disruptive disorders.

How do we succeed in silencing this draining, often-negative, fear-driven, and incessant mind-chatter? In *Think, Learn, and Succeed*, we are given a message of practical hope that a scientifically based, practically applied, and result-achievable program of action is in our hands.

Each chapter addressing an essential mindset is emphatically positive and practical, and the associated "activation tips" bring the information to practical application with a few simple steps, which ultimately can sprout real success, manifesting in a changing life.

With the foundational understanding of our own unique ways of thinking, feeling, and choosing, reflected through our mindsets, our "customized" thinking is further uniquely manifested through our individualized giftedness. With this being clarified through the Gift Profile, an invaluable tool to understand our seven modules of thinking, we have an experiential clarification of our own cycles of thought.

Finally (and, I find, one of the most important elements of each of Dr. Leaf's books), is the Recommended Reading. This last and often overlooked portion is of immense value. It documents the scientific foundations, evidence base, and sound wisdom of all of Dr. Leaf's works—and serves as an extensive bibliography and thorough reference section.

Each chapter and section of *Think, Learn, Succeed* is waiting to be minded for those wishing to go deeper toward a life of living with a freed, peaceful, and healthy mind.

Robert P. Turner, MD, MSCR, QEEGD, BCN, neurologist

Appendix

Here are fourteen examples of Metacogs to show you what they can look like. I hope they stimulate you to make your own Metacogs!

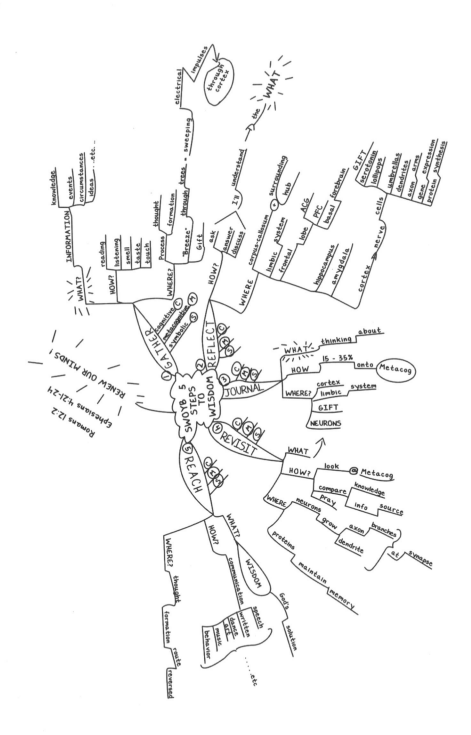

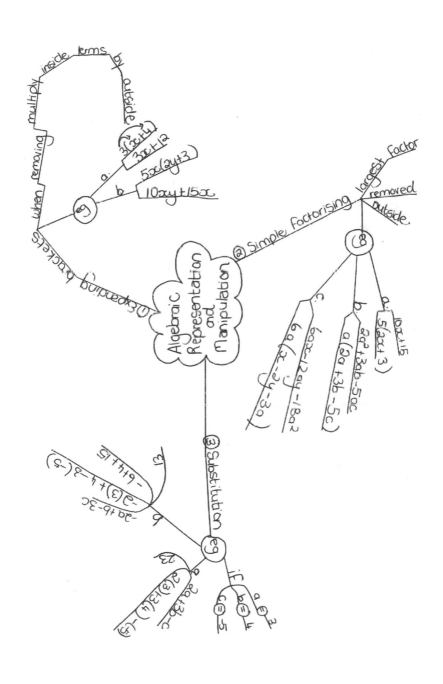

Algebraic Representation and Manipulation

① Removing brackets

when removing multiply inside terms by outside

a. $3(x+4)$
$3x+12$

b. $5x(2y+3)$
$10xy+15x$

② Simple Factorising

largest factor removed outside

a. $10x+15$
$5(2x+3)$

b. $2a^2+3ab-5ac$
$a(2a+3b-5c)$

c. $6ax-12ay-18a^2$
$6a(x-2y-3a)$

③ Substitution

eg

a $a=3$
b $b=4$
c $c=-5$

if

$3a+3b-c$
$3(3)+3(4)-(-5)$
23

$-3a+b-3c$
$-3(3)+4-3(-5)$
$-9+4+15$

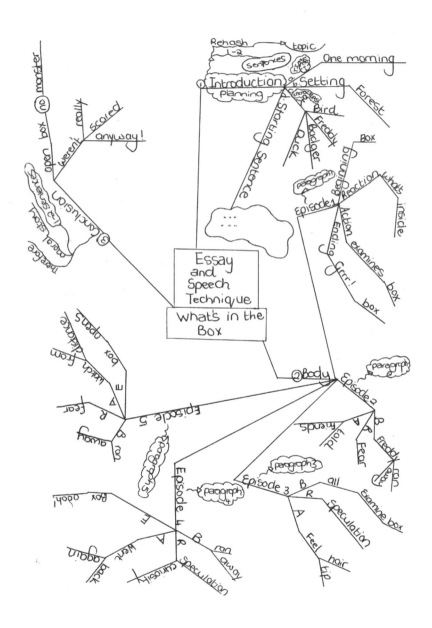

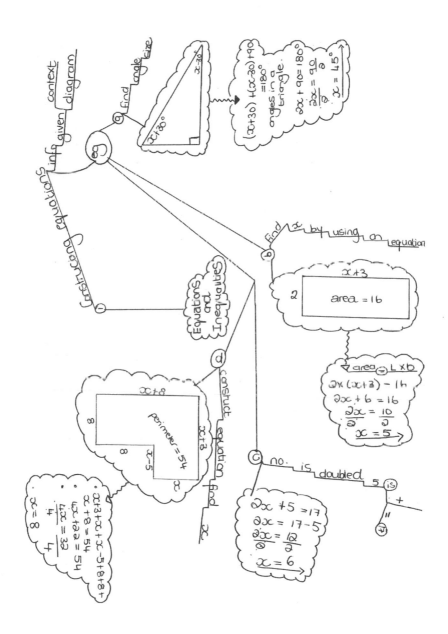

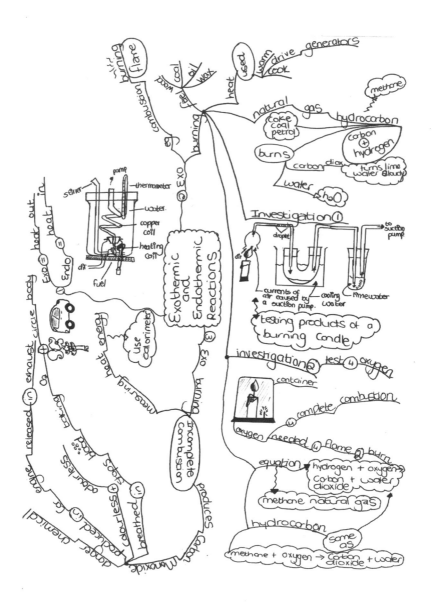

Exothermic and Endothermic Reactions

burning
air flame
peat wood coal oil wax
combustion

heat
warm drive generators
used cook

methane
natural gas hydrocarbon
coke coal petrol
burns carbon
+ hydrogen
carbon diox turns lime water cloudy
water h₂0

burning Exo 3 ©

pump
stirrer thermometer
water
copper coil
heating coil
air
fuel

Exo ≡ heat out
Endo ≡ heat in ≡

exhaust circle body
O₂
burns
food stores
colourless +
odourless
released in
breathed in
by

deadly chemical
produced (4)
Carbon
Monoxide
produces
Incomplete Combustion

measuring heat energy 12
Use calorimeter
burning exo 3

Investigation ①
droplet
air
currents of air caused by a suction pump.
cooling water
limewater
to suction pump

testing products of a burning candle

investigation ② test ④ oxygen

container
complete combustion
oxygen needed ④ flame burn
equation hydrogen + oxygen → carbon + water dioxide
methane natural gas
hydrocarbon same as
methane + oxygen → carbon dioxide + water

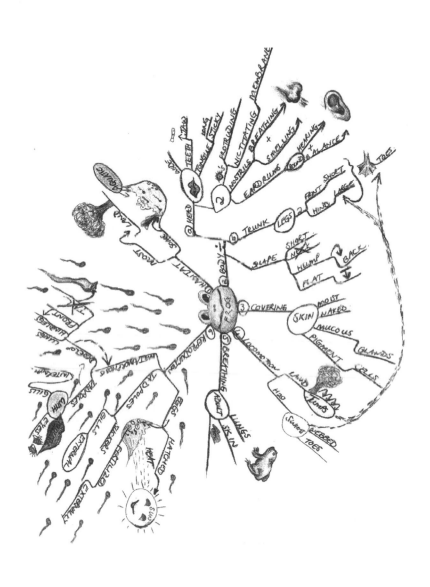

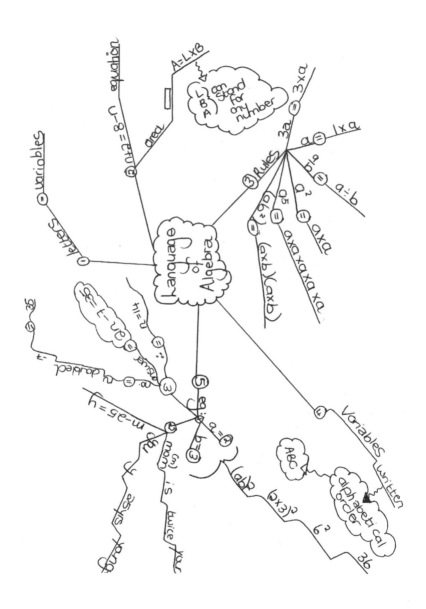

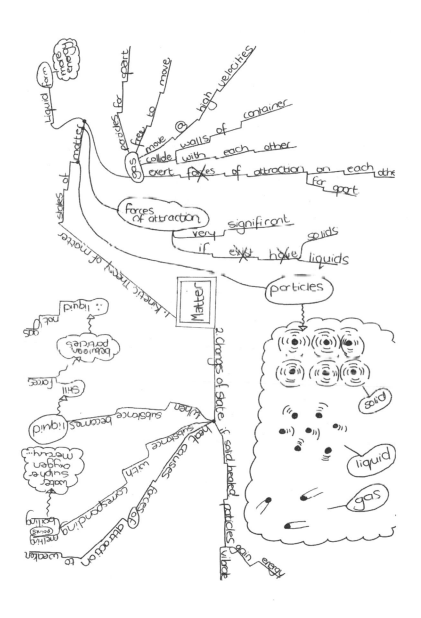

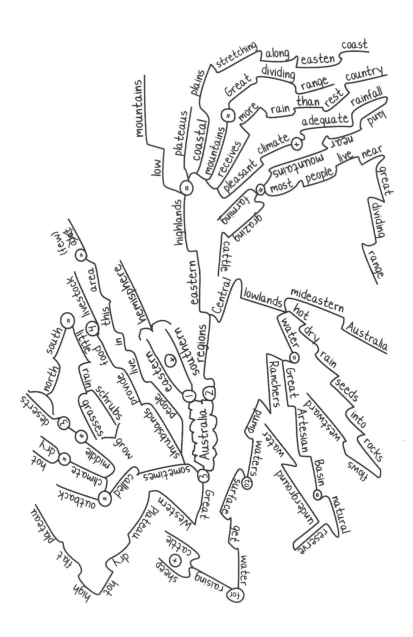

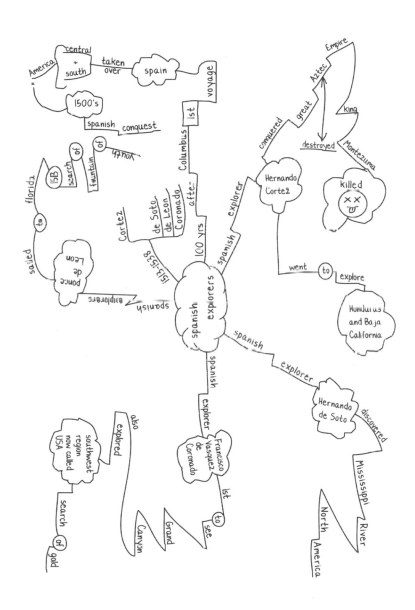

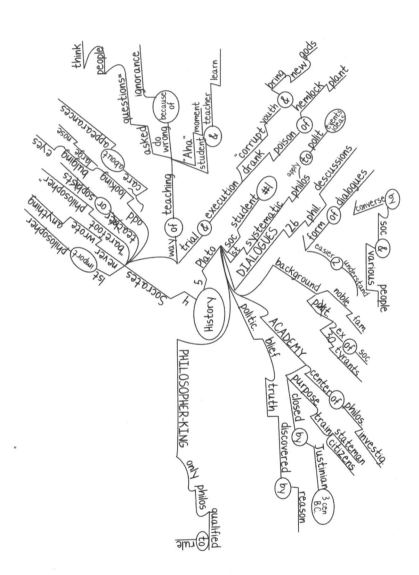

think
people
questions=
ignorance
because of
asked
"Aha" moment
do wrong
student & teacher
learn
way of teaching
looking building
odd
care about appearances
eyes
large nose
"barefoot philosopher"
"teacher of sophists"
never wrote anything
1st import. philosopher

Socrates

History

5
4

Plato
soc. student #1
trial & execution
drank poison of hemlock
plant
corrupt youth & bring new gods

apply to polit. events/ideas
philos. descussions
systematic
DIALOGUES
26 phil.
form of dialogues
converse by
soc & various people
easier 2 understand

background
noble fam.
part of soc.
ex of soc.
30 tyrants

ACADEMY
center of philos. investig.
purpose train citizens
statesman
closed by
Justinian
3 cen B.C.

politic. blief
truth
discovered by
reason

PHILOSOPHER-KING
only philos qualified to rule

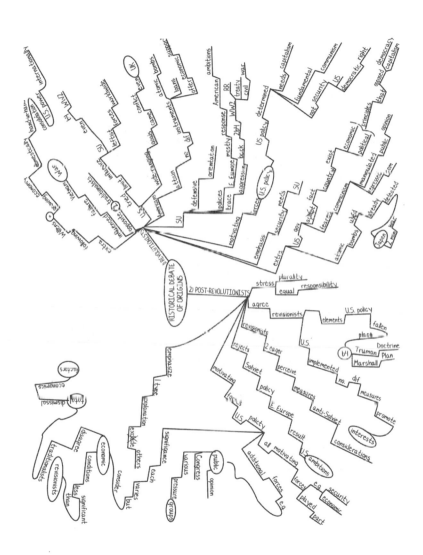

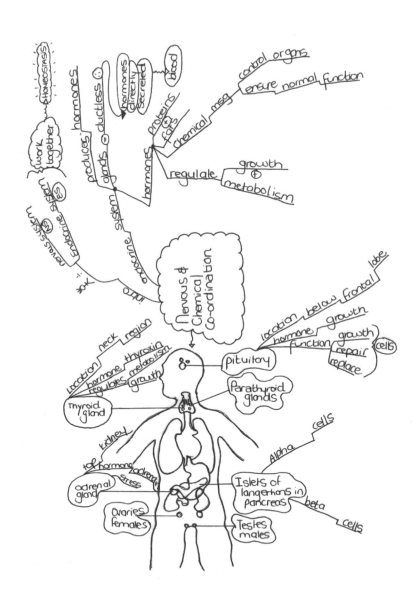

Nervous & Chemical Co-ordination

homeostasis
work together
produces hormones
endocrine system gland
nervous system work
sex
info

hormones directly secreted → blood
system glands = ductless
hormones
proteins fats ⊕
chemical msg — control organs
ensure normal function
regulate — growth ⊕ metabolism

pituitary — location below frontal lobe
hormone function — growth
growth repair replace — cells

Parathyroid glands

thyroid gland
location — neck region
hormone — thyroxin
regulates metabolism growth

kidney
total hormone adrenal stress
adrenal gland

Islets of langerhans in pancreas
Alpha cells
beta cells

ovaries females

Testes males

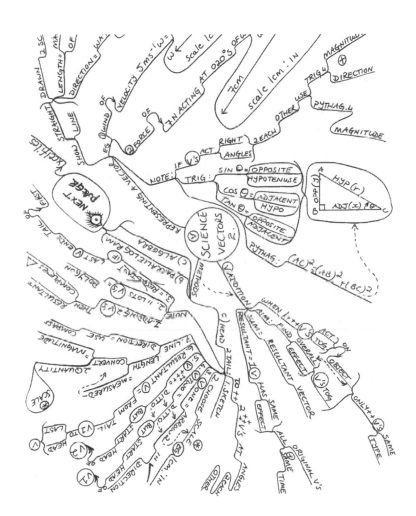

Notes

Prologue

1. Caroline Leaf, *The Perfect You: A Blueprint for Identity* (Grand Rapids: Baker Books, 2017).

Introduction Are You Succeeding or Just Surviving?

1. Julianne Holt-Lunstad et al., "Loneliness and Social Isolation as Risk Factors for Mortality: A Meta-Analytic Review," *Perspectives on Psychological Science* 10, no. 2 (2015): 227–37; Stephanie Cacioppo et al., "Loneliness: Clinical Import and Interventions," *Perspectives on Psychological Science* 10, no. 2 (2015): 238–49; Ye Luo et al., "Loneliness, Health, and Mortality in Old Age: A National Longitudinal Study," *Social Science & Medicine* 74, no. 6 (2012): 907–14; Yang Claire Yang et al., "Social Relationships and Physiological Determinants of Longevity across the Human Life Span," *Proceedings of the National Academy of Sciences* 113, no. 3 (2016): 578–83.

2. Philip Hickey, "ADHD: A Destructive Psychiatric Hoax," *Mad in America*, October 30, 2016, https://www.madinamerica.com/2016/10/adhd-destructive-psychiatric -hoax/; S. P. Hinshaw and R. M. Scheffler, *The ADHD Explosion: Myths, Medication, Money, and Today's Push for Performance* (New York: Oxford University Press, 2014).

3. Eric Maisel, "Future of Mental Health Interview Series: Interview with Joanna Moncrieff on the Myth of the Medical Cure," *Mad in America*, February 15, 2016, https://www.madinamerica.com/2016/02/future-of-mental-health-interview-series -interview-with-joanna-moncrieff-on-the-myth-of-the-chemical-cure/.

4. P. Kinderman, *A Prescription for Psychiatry: Why We Need a Whole New Approach to Mental Health and Wellbeing* (London: Palgrave Macmillan, 2014); P. Kinderman, *New Laws of Psychology: Why Nature and Nurture Alone Can't Explain Human Behaviour* (London: Constable & Robinson, 2014).

5. Carl Benedikt Frey and Michael A. Osborne, "The Future of Employment: How Susceptible Are Jobs to Computerisation?" *Technological Forecasting and Social Change* 114 (2017): 254–80.

6. Andi Horvath, "How Does Technology Affect Our Brains?" *The Age*, June 4, 2015, http://www.theage.com.au/national/education/voice/how-does-technology-affect-our-brains-20150604-3x5uq.html; Cornell University, "Chances Are You Don't Remember What You Just Retweeted: Experiments Show 'Retweeting' Can Interfere with Learning and Memory, Both Online and Off," *ScienceDaily*, April 29, 2016, www.sciencedaily.com/releases/2016/04/160429095028.htm; Davide Ponzi et al., "Cortisol, Salivary Alpha-amylase and Children's Perceptions of Their Social Networks," *Social Neuroscience* 11, no. 2 (2016): 164–74; Bernard McCoy, "Digital Distractions in the Classroom: Student Classroom Use of Digital Devices for Non-Class Related Purposes," *Journal of Media Education*, October 15, 2013; Jeffrey H. Kuznekoff, Stevie Munz, and Scott Titsworth, "Mobile Phones in the Classroom: Examining the Effects of Texting, Twitter, and Message Content on Student Learning," *Communication Education* 64, no. 3 (2015): 344–65; "Digital Media May Be Changing How You Think," *Dartmouth Press Releases*, May 8, 2016, https://www.dartmouth.edu/press-releases/digital-media-change-050816.html; Daniel B. le Roux and Douglas A. Parry, "In-Lecture Media Use and Academic Performance: Does Subject Area Matter?" *Computers in Human Behavior* 77 (2017): 86–94; Stephen Houghton et al., "Virtually Impossible: Limiting Australian Children and Adolescents Daily Screen Based Media Use," *BMC Public Health* 15, no. 1 (2015): 5; Andrew K. Przybylski and Netta Weinstein, "A Large-Scale Test of the Goldilocks Hypothesis: Quantifying the Relations between Digital-Screen Use and the Mental Well-being of Adolescents," *Psychological Science* 28, no. 2 (2017): 204–15; Hayley Christian et al., "Nowhere to Go and Nothing to Do but Sit? Youth Screen Time and the Association with Access to Neighborhood Destinations," *Environment and Behavior* 49, no. 1 (2017): 84–108; Kep Kee Loh and Ryota Kanai, "Higher Media Multi-tasking Activity Is Associated with Smaller Gray-matter Density in the Anterior Cingulate Cortex," *PloS One* 9, no. 9 (2014): e106698.

7. Ibid.

8. Tony Schwartz and Christine Porath, "Why You Hate Work," *New York Times*, May 30, 2014, https://www.nytimes.com/2014/06/01/opinion/sunday/why-you-hate-work.html.

9. Rutger Bregman, "Poverty Isn't a Lack of Character; It's a Lack of Cash," TED video, recorded April 2017 at TED2017, 13:59, https://www.ted.com/talks/rutger_bregman_poverty_isn_t_a_lack_of_character_it_s_a_lack_of_cash/transcript.

10. Paul A. Howard-Jones, "Neuroscience and Education: Myths and Messages," *Nature Reviews Neuroscience* 15, no. 12 (2014): 817–24; Daniel T. Willingham, Elizabeth M. Hughes, and David G. Dobolyi, "The Scientific Status of Learning Styles Theories," *Teaching of Psychology* 42, no. 3 (2015): 266–71; Sanne Dekker et al., "Neuromyths in Education: Prevalence and Predictors of Misconceptions Among Teachers," *Frontiers in Psychology* 3 (2012); Philip M. Newton, "The Learning Styles Myth Is Thriving in Higher Education," *Frontiers in Psychology* 6 (2015); John Geake, "Neuromythologies in Education," *Educational Research* 50, no. 2 (2008): 123–33; Universiteit Leiden, "A Philosophical Mythbuster," *ScienceDaily*, accessed November 18, 2017, www.sciencedaily.com/releases/2017/08/170831093239.htm; Patricia Wolfe, "Brain-Compatible Learning: Fad or Foundation? Neuroscience Points to Better Strategies for Educators,

but Sorting Out Claims on Brain-Based Programs Is Essential," *School Administrator* 63, no. 11 (2006): 10–16; Christian Jarrett, *Great Myths of the Brain* (Hoboken, NJ: Wiley, 2014); Anthony M. Grant, "Coaching the Brain: Neuro-Science or Neuro-Nonsense," *The Coaching Psychologist* 11, no. 1 (2015): 31; Sebastiano Massaro, "Neurofeedback in the Workplace: From Neurorehabilitation Hope to Neuroleadership Hype?" *International Journal of Rehabilitation Research* 38, no. 3 (2015): 276–78; Lisa Carey, "Neuromyths and the Classroom," *Linking Research to Classrooms*, August 18, 2015, https://www.kennedykrieger.org/professional-training/training-disciplines/special-education-fellowship/linking-research-classrooms-blog/neuromyths-classroom.

11. Kelly Macdonald et al., "Dispelling the Myth: Training in Education or Neuroscience Decreases but Does Not Eliminate Beliefs in Neuromyths," *Frontiers in Psychology* 8 (2017): 1314.

12. Ibid.

13. Xaq Pitkow and Dora E. Angelaki, "Inference in the Brain: Statistics Flowing in Redundant Population Codes," *Neuron* 94, no. 5 (2017): 943–53; Rice University, "Simple Tasks Don't Test Brain's True Complexity," *ScienceDaily*, www.sciencedaily.com/releases/2017/06/170608133355.htm.

14. Macdonald et al., "Dispelling the Myth."

15. Caroline Leaf, "The Mind Mapping Approach: A Model and Framework for Geodesic Learning," unpublished DPhil dissertation, University of Pretoria, South Africa, 1997.

16. Tyler L. Harrison et al., "Working Memory Training May Increase Working Memory Capacity but Not Fluid Intelligence," *Psychological Science* 24, no. 12 (2013): 2409–19; Thomas S. Redick et al., "No Evidence of Intelligence Improvement After Working Memory Training: A Randomized, Placebo-Controlled Study," *Journal of Experimental Psychology: General* 142, no. 2 (2013): 359; Weng-Tink Chooi and Lee A. Thompson, "Working Memory Training Does Not Improve Intelligence in Healthy Young Adults," *Intelligence* 40, no. 6 (2012): 531–42.

17. Daniel J. Simons et al., "Do 'Brain-Training' Programs Work?" *Psychological Science in the Public Interest* 17, no. 3 (2016): 103–86; Dustin J. Souders et al., "Evidence for Narrow Transfer after Short-Term Cognitive Training in Older Adults," *Frontiers in Aging Neuroscience* 9 (2017); Sheida Rabipour et al., "What Do People Expect of Cognitive Enhancement?" *Journal of Cognitive Enhancement* (2017): 1–8; Pauline L. Baniqued et al., "Working Memory, Reasoning, and Task Switching Training: Transfer Effects, Limitations, and Great Expectations?" *PloS One* 10, no. 11 (2015): e0142169; Cyrus K. Foroughi et al., "Placebo Effects in Cognitive Training," *Proceedings of the National Academy of Sciences* 113, no. 27 (2016): 7470–74; Monica Melby-Lervåg and Charles Hulme, "Is Working Memory Training Effective? A Meta-Analytic Review," *Developmental Psychology* 49, no. 2 (2013): 270; D. M. Curlik and T. J. Shors, "Training Your Brain: Do Mental and Physical (MAP) Training Enhance Cognition through the Process of Neurogenesis in the Hippocampus?" *Neuropharmacology* 64 (2013): 506–14.

18. Curlik and Shors, "Training Your Brain."

19. Monica Melby-Lervåg, Thomas S. Redick, and Charles Hulme, "Working Memory Training Does Not Improve Performance on Measures of Intelligence or Other Measures of 'Far Transfer' Evidence from a Meta-Analytic Review," *Perspectives on Psychological Science* 11, no. 4 (2016): 512–34.; Simons et al., "Do 'Brain-Training' Programs Work?"; Matthias Schwaighofer, Frank Fischer, and Markus Bühner, "Does

Working Memory Training Transfer? A Meta-Analysis including Training Conditions as Moderators," *Educational Psychologist* 50, no. 2 (2015): 138–66.

20. Ibid.

21. Leaf, "The Mind Mapping Approach."

22. Caroline Leaf, "Mind Mapping: A Therapeutic Technique for Closed Head Injury," master's dissertation, University of Pretoria, South Africa, 1990; Caroline Leaf, "An Altered Perception of Learning: Geodesic Learning: Part 2," *Therapy Africa* 2, no. 1 (January/February 1998): 4; C. M. Leaf, "An Altered Perception of Learning: Geodesic Learning," *Therapy Africa* 1 (October 1997): 7; Leaf, *The Perfect You*; Caroline Leaf, "Teaching Children to Make the Most of Their Minds: Mind Mapping," *Journal for Technical and Vocational Education in South Africa* 121 (1990): 11–13; Caroline Leaf, *Switch On Your Brain: Understand Your Unique Intelligence Profile and Maximize Your Potential* (Cape Town, South Africa: Tafelberg, 2005).

Chapter 1 Thinking and Learning to Succeed

1. Ulrich W. Weger and Stephen Loughnan, "Mobilizing Unused Resources: Using the Placebo Concept to Enhance Cognitive Performance," *The Quarterly Journal of Experimental Psychology* 66, no. 1 (2013): 23–28; B. Lipton, *The Biology of Belief: Unleashing the Power of Consciousness, Matter and Miracles* (Santa Cruz, CA: Mountain of Love Productions, 2008); Fabrizio Benedetti, "Placebo Effects: From the Neurobiological Paradigm to Translational Implications," *Neuron* 84, no. 3 (2014): 623–37; Michael B. Steinborn, Robert Langner, and Lynn Huestegge, "Mobilizing Cognition for Speeded Action: Try-Harder Instructions Promote Motivated Readiness in the Constant-Foreperiod Paradigm," *Psychological Research* 81, no. 6 (2017): 1135–51; Sophie Parker et al., "A Sham Drug Improves a Demanding Prospective Memory Task," *Memory* 19, no. 6 (2011): 606–12; Danielle Adams, "Exploring the Attentional Processes of Expert Performers and the Impact of Priming on Motor Skill Execution," PhD dissertation, Brunel University School of Sport and Education, 2010; Ulrich W. Weger and Stephen Loughnan, "Using Participant Choice to Enhance Memory Performance," *Applied Cognitive Psychology* 29, no. 3 (2015): 345–49; Ellen J. Langer, *Counter Clockwise: Mindful Health and the Power of Possibility* (New York: Ballantine, 2009).

2. Ibid.

3. Lynne McTaggart, *The Intention Experiment: Using Your Thoughts to Change Your Life and the World* (New York: Atria, 2008), Kindle loc. 160–61.

4. McTaggart, *Intention Experiment*; William W. Monafo and Michael A. West, "Current Treatment Recommendations for Topical Burn Therapy," *Drugs* 40, no. 3 (1990): 364–73; Alia J. Crum and Ellen J. Langer, "Mind-Set Matters: Exercise and the Placebo Effect," *Psychological Science* 18, no. 2 (2007): 165–71; Shawn Achor, *The Happiness Advantage: The Seven Principles of Positive Psychology That Fuel Success and Performance at Work* (New York: Random House, 2011); Alia J. Crum, Peter Salovey, and Shawn Achor, "Rethinking Stress: the Role of Mindsets in Determining the Stress Response," *Journal of Personality and Social Psychology* 104, no. 4 (2013): 716; Alia J. Crum et al., "Mind over Milkshakes: Mindsets, Not Just Nutrients, Determine Ghrelin Response," *Health Psychology* 30, no. 4 (2011): 424; Justin M. Berg, Jane E. Dutton, and Amy Wrzesniewski, "Job Crafting and Meaningful Work," *Purpose and Meaning in the Workplace* (2013): 81–104; Alison Wood Brooks, "Get Excited: Reappraising

Pre-Performance Anxiety as Excitement," *Journal of Experimental Psychology: General* 143, no. 3 (2014): 1144; Andrew R. Todd et al., "Anxious and Egocentric: How Specific Emotions Influence Perspective Taking," *Journal of Experimental Psychology: General* 144, no. 2 (2015): 374; Jiyoung Park, Özlem Ayduk, and Ethan Kross, "Stepping Back to Move Forward: Expressive Writing Promotes Self-Distancing," *Emotion* 16, no. 3 (2016): 349; Miranda L. Beltzer et al., "Rethinking Butterflies: The Affective, Physiological, and Performance Effects of Reappraising Arousal During Social Evaluation," *Emotion* 14, no. 4 (2014): 761; Jeremy P. Jamieson, Wendy Berry Mendes, and Matthew K. Nock, "Improving Acute Stress Responses: The Power of Reappraisal," *Current Directions in Psychological Science* 22, no. 1 (2013): 51–56; Jeremy P. Jamieson et al., "Turning the Knots in Your Stomach into Bows: Reappraising Arousal Improves Performance on the GRE," *Journal of Experimental Social Psychology* 46, no. 1 (2010): 208–12.

5. Fabrizio Benedetti et al., "When Words Are Painful: Unraveling the Mechanisms of the Nocebo Effect," *Neuroscience* 147, no. 2 (2007): 260–71; Fabrizio Benedetti et al., "The Biochemical and Neuroendocrine Bases of the Hyperalgesic Nocebo Effect," *Journal of Neuroscience* 26, no. 46 (2006): 12014–22; Luana Colloca, Monica Sigaudo, and Fabrizio Benedetti, "The Role of Learning in Nocebo and Placebo Effects," *Pain* 136, no. 1 (2008): 211–18; L. Horsfall, "The Nocebo Effect," *SAAD digest* 32 (2016): 55–57; Jian Kong et al., "A Functional Magnetic Resonance Imaging Study on the Neural Mechanisms of Hyperalgesic Nocebo Effect," *Journal of Neuroscience* 28, no. 49 (2008): 13354–62.

6. Fabrizio Benedetti, Elisa Carlino, and Antonella Pollo, "How Placebos Change the Patient's Brain," *Neuropsychopharmacology* 36, no. 1 (2011): 339–54; Helen E. Fisher et al., "Reward, Addiction, and Emotion Regulation Systems Associated with Rejection in Love," *Journal of Neurophysiology* 104, no. 1 (2010): 51–60; Xiaomeng Xu et al., "Reward and Motivation Systems: A Brain Mapping Study of Early-Stage Intense Romantic Love in Chinese Participants," *Human Brain Mapping* 32, no. 2 (2011): 249–57; Bianca P. Acevedo et al., "Neural Correlates of Long-Term Intense Romantic Love," *Social Cognitive and Affective Neuroscience* 7, no. 2 (2012): 145–59.

7. Benedetti, Carlino, and Pollo, "How Placebos Change the Patient's Brain;" McTaggart, *Intention Experiment*; William W. Monafo and Michael A. West, "Current Treatment Recommendations for Topical Burn Therapy," *Drugs* 40, no. 3 (1990): 364–73; Crum and Langer, "Mind-Set Matters;" Achor, *Happiness Advantage*; Crum, Salovey, and Achor, "Rethinking Stress;" Crum et al., "Mind over Milkshakes;" Berg, Dutton, and Wrzesniewski, "Job Crafting and Meaningful Work;" Brooks, "Get Excited;" Todd et al., "Anxious and Egocentric;" Park, Ayduk, and Kross, "Stepping Back to Move Forward;" Beltzer et al., "Rethinking Butterflies."

8. Jamieson, Mendes, and Nock, "Improving Acute Stress Responses."

9. H. P. Stapp, "Quantum Interactive-Dualism: An Alternative to Materialism," *Journal of Religion and Science* 3 (2006), doi:10.1111/j.1467–9744.2005.00762.x, http://www-atlas.lbl.gov/~stapp/QID.pdf.

10. Brooks, "Get Excited."

11. Mona Dekoven Fishbane, "Wired to Connect: Neuroscience, Relationships, and Therapy," *Family Process* 46, no. 3 (2007): 395–412; Stan Tatkin, *Wired for Love: How Understanding Your Partner's Brain and Attachment Style Can Help You Defuse Conflict and Build a Secure Relationship* (Oakland, CA: New Harbinger, 2012); Mona DeKoven Fishbane, *Loving with the Brain in Mind: Neurobiology and Couple Therapy*

(New York: Norton, 2013); Tali Sharot et al., "Neural Mechanisms Mediating Optimism Bias," *Nature* 450, no. 7166 (2007): 102–5; Tali Sharot, "The Optimism Bias," *Current Biology* 21, no. 23 (2011): R941–45; Iain Chalmers and Robert Matthews, "What Are the Implications of Optimism Bias in Clinical Research?" *The Lancet* 367, no. 9509 (2006): 449–50; Tali Sharot, *The Optimism Bias: A Tour of the Irrationally Positive Brain* (New York: Vintage, 2011); Neil D. Weinstein, "Unrealistic Optimism about Future Life Events," *Journal of Personality and Social Psychology* 39, no. 5 (1980): 806; B. H. Lipton, "Insight into Cellular Consciousness," *Bridges* 12, no. 1 (2012): 5; B. H. Lipton, *The Biology of Belief: Unleashing the Power of Consciousness* (Santa Rosa, CA: Mountain of Love/Elite Books, 2005); Leaf, *Switch On Your Brain*; Caroline Leaf, "21-Day Brain Detox," www. 21daybraindetox.com; Leaf, *The Perfect You*; E. B. Raposa, H. B. Laws, and E. B. Ansell, "Prosocial Behavior Mitigates the Negative Effects of Stress in Everyday Life," *Clinical Psychological Science* (2015), doi:10.1177/2167702615611073; Dawson Church, *The Genie in Your Genes: Epigenetic Medicine and the New Science of Intention* (Santa Rosa, CA: Energy Psychology Press, 2009); Stanton Peele and Archie Brodsky, *Love and Addiction* (New York: Taplinger, 1975); Stanton Peele, "The 7 Hardest Addictions to Quit—Love is the Worst," *Psychology Today*, December 15, 2008, https://www.psychologytoday.com/blog/addiction -in-society/200812/the-7-hardest-addictions-quit-love-is-the-worst; Tatkin, *Wired for Love*; E. R. Kandel, *In Search of Memory: The Emergence of a New Science of Mind* (New York: Norton, 2008).

12. Alex Paul, Zayna Chaker, and Fiona Doetsch, "Hypothalamic Regulation of Regionally Distinct Adult Neural Stem Cells and Neurogenesis," *Science* (2017): eaal3839; Julia P. Andreotti et al., "Hypothalamic Neurons Take Center Stage in the Neural Stem Cell Niche," *Cell Stem Cell* 21, no. 3 (2017): 293–94; T. J. Shors et al., "Use It or Lose It: How Neurogenesis Keeps the Brain Fit for Learning," *Behavioural Brain Research* 227, no. 2 (2012): 450–58; Daniel M. Curlik and Tracey J. Shors, "Learning Increases the Survival of Newborn Neurons Provided That Learning Is Difficult to Achieve and Successful," *Journal of Cognitive Neuroscience* 23, no. 9 (2011): 2159–70; Megan L. Anderson et al., "Associative Learning Increases Adult Neurogenesis During a Critical Period," *European Journal of Neuroscience* 33, no. 1 (2011): 175–81; Gina DiFeo and Tracey J. Shors, "Mental and Physical Skill Training Increases Neurogenesis via Cell Survival in the Adolescent Hippocampus," *Brain Research* 1654 (2017): 95–101; Michael A. Bonaguidi et al., "In Vivo Clonal Analysis Reveals Self-Renewing and Multipotent Adult Neural Stem Cell Characteristics," *Cell* 145, no. 7 (2011): 1142–55.

13. Shors et al., "Use It or Lose It."

14. Alex Paul, Chaker, and Doetsch, "Hypothalamic Regulation."

15. Fuzheng Guo et al., "Pyramidal Neurons Are Generated from Oligodendroglial Progenitor Cells in Adult Piriform Cortex," *Journal of Neuroscience* 30, no. 36 (2010): 12036–49; Azad Bonni et al., "Regulation of Gliogenesis in the Central Nervous System by the JAK-STAT Signaling Pathway," *Science* 278, no. 5337 (1997): 477–83; Shama Bansod, Ryoichiro Kageyama, and Toshiyuki Ohtsuka, "Hes5 Regulates the Transition Timing of Neurogenesis and Gliogenesis in Mammalian Neocortical Development," *Development* 144, no. 17 (2017): 3156–67; Sarah Jäkel and Leda Dimou, "Glial Cells and Their Function in the Adult Brain: A Journey through the History of Their Ablation," *Frontiers in Cellular Neuroscience* 11 (2017).

16. Dan G. Blazer and Lyla M. Hernandez, eds., *Genes, Behavior, and the Social Environment: Moving Beyond the Nature/Nurture Debate* (Washington, DC: National Academies Press, 2006); David C. Witherington and Robert Lickliter, "Transcending the Nature-Nurture Debate through Epigenetics: Are We There Yet?" *Human Development* 60, no. 2–3 (2017): 65–68; Katherine Weatherford Darling et al., "Enacting the Molecular Imperative: How Gene-Environment Interaction Research Links Bodies and Environments in the Post-Genomic Age," *Social Science & Medicine* 155 (2016): 51–60; Bruce H. Lipton, *The Biology of Belief* (New York: Hay House, 2008) Kindle loc. 115ff.; Dawson Church, *The Genie in Your Genes: Epigenetic Medicine and the New Biology of Intention* (Santa Rosa, CA: Energy Psychology Press, 2009); Antonei B. Csoka and Moshe Szyf, "Epigenetic Side-Effects of Common Pharmaceuticals: A Potential New Field in Medicine and Pharmacology," *Medical Hypotheses* 73, no. 5 (2009): 770–80; Maurizio Meloni and Giuseppe Testa, "Scrutinizing the Epigenetics Revolution," *BioSocieties* 9, no. 4 (2014): 431–56; Cosmas D. Arnold et al., "Genome-Wide Quantitative Enhancer Activity Maps Identified by STARR=Seq," *Science* 339, no. 6123 (March 1, 2013): 1074–77; L. I. Patrushev and T. F. Kovalenko, "Functions of Noncoding Sequences in Mammalian Genomes," *Biochemistry* (Mosc.) 79, no. 13 (December 2014): 1442–69; Manolis Kellis et al., "Defining Functional DNA Elements in the Human Genome," *Proc Natl Acad Sci USA* 111, no. 17 (April 29, 2014): 6131–38; Perla Kaliman et al., "Rapid Changes in Histone Deacetylases and Inflammatory Gene Expression in Expert Meditators," *Psychoneuroendocrinology* 40 (February 2014): 96–107; Robin Holliday, "Epigenetics: A Historical Overview," *Epigenetics* 1, no. 2 (2006): 76–80; Adrian Bird, "Perceptions of Epigenetics," *Nature* 447, no. 7143 (2007): 396398; J. J. Day and J. D. Sweatt, "Epigenetic Mechanisms in Cognition," *Neuron* 70, no. 5 (2011): 813–29 ; Trygve Tollefsbol, ed., *Handbook of Epigenetics: The New Molecular and Medical Genetics* (New York: Elsevier/Academic Press, 2011), Bob Weinhold, "Epigenetics: The Science of Change," *Environmental Health Perspectives* 114, no. 3 (2006): A160; John Cairns, Julie Overbaugh, and Stephan Miller, "The Origin of Mutants," *Nature* 335 (1988): 142–45; H. F. Nijhout, "Metaphors and the Role of Genes in Development," *Bioessays* 12, no. 9 (1990): 441–46; Leaf, *The Perfect You*, Kindle loc. 3296–305.

17. Ibid.

18. Ibid.

19. Ibid.

20. Deirdre A. Robertson and Rose Anne Kenny, "Negative Perceptions of Aging Modify the Association between Frailty and Cognitive Function in Older Adults," *Personality and Individual Differences* 100 (2016): 120–25; Susanne Wurm et al., "How Do Views on Aging Affect Health Outcomes in Adulthood and Late Life? Explanations for an Established Connection," *Developmental Review* (2017).

21. Patrick L. Hill, Grant W. Edmonds, and Sarah E. Hampson, "A Purposeful Lifestyle Is a Healthful Lifestyle: Linking Sense of Purpose to Self-Rated Health through Multiple Health Behaviors," *Journal of Health Psychology* (2017): 1–9.

22. Caroline Leaf, *Think and Eat Yourself Smart* (Grand Rapids: Baker Books, 2016).

23. Nicolas Cherbuin et al., "Validated Alzheimer's Disease Risk Index (ANU-ADRI) Is Associated with Smaller Volumes in the Default Mode Network in the Early 60s," *Brain Imaging and Behavior* (2017): 1–10.

24. Suzanne C. Segerstrom, "Optimism and Immunity: Do Positive Thoughts Always Lead to Positive Effects?" *Brain, Behavior, and Immunity* 19, no. 3 (2005): 195–200; Fishbane, "Wired to Connect;" Tatkin, *Wired for Love*; Fishbane, *Loving with the Brain in Mind*; Sharot, *The Optimism Bias.*

25. Ibid.

26. Leaf, *Switch On Your Brain.*

27. Leaf, *Switch On Your Brain*; Leaf, *The Perfect You*; Leaf, *Think and Eat Yourself Smart*; Segerstrom, "Optimism and Immunity;" Diana Gruia and Andreea Munteanu, "Optimism in Daily Life," *Communicating Across Cultures*: 49; Suzanne C. Segerstrom, Iana Boggero, and Daniel R. Evans, "Pause and Plan," *Handbook of Self-Regulation: Research, Theory, and Applications* (2017): 131; Anne Böckler, Anita Tusche, and Tania Singer, "The Structure of Human Prosociality: Differentiating Altruistically Motivated, Norm Motivated, Strategically Motivated, and Self-Reported Prosocial Behavior," *Social Psychological and Personality Science* 7, no. 6 (2016): 530–41; Anita Tusche et al., "Decoding the Charitable Brain: Empathy, Perspective Taking, and Attention Shifts Differentially Predict Altruistic Giving," *Journal of Neuroscience* 36, no. 17 (2016): 4719–32; Indrajeet Patil et al., "Neuroanatomical Basis of Concern-Based Altruism in Virtual Environment," *Neuropsychologia* (2017); Jacek Debiec and Andreas Olsson, "Social Fear Learning: From Animal Models to Human Function," *Trends in Cognitive Sciences* (2017); Siobhan S. Pattwell and Kevin G. Bath, "Emotional Learning, Stress, and Development: An Ever-Changing Landscape Shaped by Early-Life Experience," *Neurobiology of Learning and Memory* (2017); Andreas Olsson and Elizabeth A. Phelps, "Social Learning of Fear," *Nature Neuroscience* 10, no. 9 (2007): 1095–102.

28. Ibid.

29. C. M. Leaf, I. C. Uys, and B. Louw, "An Alternative Non-Traditional Approach to Learning: The Metacognitive-Mapping Approach," *The South African Journal of Communication Disorders* 45 (1998): 87–102; C. M. Leaf, I. C. Uys, and B. Louw, "The Development of a Model for Geodesic Learning: The Geodesic Information Processing Model," *The South African Journal of Communication Disorders* 44 (1997): 53–70; C. M. Leaf, I. C. Uys, and B. Louw, "The Mind Mapping Approach (MMA): A Culture and Language-Free Technique," *The South African Journal of Communication Disorders* 40 (1992): 35–43; Leaf, "The Mind Mapping Approach," unpublished DPhil dissertation; C. M. Leaf, I. C. Uys, and B. Louw, "Mind Mapping as a Therapeutic Intervention Technique," unpublished workshop manual, 1985; C. M. Leaf, I. C. Uys, and B. Louw, "Mind Mapping as a Therapeutic Technique," *Communiphon* 296 (1989): 11–15.

Chapter 2 The Thinker Mindset

1. American Psychological Association, "Stress in America: Coping with Change," *Stress in America™ Survey* (2017).

2. Timothy D. Wilson et al., "Which Would You Prefer—Do Nothing or Receive Electric Shocks!" *Science* 345, no. 6192 (2014): 75–77; Timothy D. Wilson et al., "Just Think: The Challenges of the Disengaged Mind," *Science* 345, no. 6192 (2014): 75–77; Martin Pielot et al., "When Attention Is Not Scarce—Detecting Boredom from Mobile Phone Usage," *Proceedings of the 2015 ACM International Joint Conference on Pervasive and Ubiquitous Computing*, 825–36; Paul Seli et al., "Mind-Wandering with and

without Intention," *Trends in Cognitive Sciences* 20, no. 8 (2016): 605–17; Russell B. Clayton, Glenn Leshner, and Anthony Almond, "The Extended iSelf: The Impact of iPhone Separation on Cognition, Emotion, and Physiology," *Journal of Computer-Mediated Communication* 20, no. 2 (2015): 119–35.

3. David Z. Morris, "Less Work, Less Sex, Less Happiness: We're Losing Generation Z to the Smartphone," *Fortune*, August 7, 2017, http://amp.timeinc.net/fortune /2017/08/06/generation-z-smartphone-depression/?source=dam; Jean M. Twenge, *Generation Me—Revised and Updated: Why Today's Young Americans Are More Confident, Assertive, Entitled—and More Miserable Than Ever Before* (New York: Atria, 2014); Jean M. Twenge et al., "Increases in Depressive Symptoms, Suicide-Related Outcomes, and Suicide Rates among US Adolescents after 2010 and Links to Increased New Media Screen Time," *Clinical Psychological Science* 6, no. 1 (2017): 3–17; Jean M. Twenge, Zlatan Krizan, and Garrett Hisler, "Decreases in Self-Reported Sleep Duration among US Adolescents 2009–2015 and Links to New Media Screen Time," *Sleep Medicine* 39 (September 2017); Pooja S. Tandon et al., "Home Environment Relationships with Children's Physical Activity, Sedentary Time, and Screen Time by Socioeconomic Status," *International Journal of Behavioral Nutrition and Physical Activity* 9, no. 1 (2012); 88, Gary Small and Gigi Vorgan, *iBrain: Surviving the Technological Alteration of the Modern Mind* (New York: HarperCollins, 2009); Ofir Turel and Hamed Qahri-Saremi, "Problematic Use of Social Networking Sites: Antecedents and Consequence from a Dual-System Theory Perspective," *Journal of Management Information Systems* 33, no. 4 (2016): 1087–116; Qinghua He et al., "Excess Social Media Use in Normal Populations Is Associated with Amygdala-Striatal but Not with Prefrontal Morphology," *Psychiatry Research: Neuroimaging* 269 (2017): 31–35; Ofir Turel et al., "Social Networking Sites Use and the Morphology of a Social-Semantic Brain Network," *Social Neuroscience* (2017): 1–9; Qinghua He, Ofir Turel, and Antoine Béchara, "Brain Anatomy Alterations Associated with Social Networking Site (SNS) Addiction," *Scientific Reports* 7 (2017): 45064.

4. Twenge, *Generation Me*; Twenge et al., "Increases in Depressive Symptoms;" Twenge, Krizan, and Hisler, "Decreases in Self-Reported Sleep Duration."

5. David Blackwell et al., "Extraversion, Neuroticism, Attachment Style and Fear of Missing Out as Predictors of Social Media Use and Addiction," *Personality and Individual Differences* 116 (2017): 69–72; Héctor Fuster, Andrés Chamarro, and Ursula Oberst, "Fear of Missing Out, Online Social Networking and Mobile Phone Addiction: A Latent Profile Approach," *Journal of Adolescence* 55 (2017); Elisa Wegmann et al., "Online-Specific Fear of Missing Out and Internet-Use Expectancies Contribute to Symptoms of Internet-Communication Disorder," *Addictive Behaviors Reports* 5 (2017): 33–42; Bobby Swar and Tahir Hameed, "Fear of Missing Out, Social Media Engagement, Smartphone Addiction and Distraction: Moderating Role of Self-Help Mobile Apps-Based Interventions in the Youth," *HEALTHINF* (2017): 139–46.

6. Christine A. Godwin et al., "Functional Connectivity within and between Intrinsic Brain Networks Correlates with Trait Mind Wandering," *Neuropsychologia* 103 (2017): 140–53.

7. Ibid.

8. Kalina Christoff et al., "Mind-Wandering as Spontaneous Thought: a Dynamic Framework," *Nature Reviews Neuroscience* 17, no. 11 (2016): 718–31.

9. Ibid.

10. Leaf, *Switch On Your Brain*; J. Paul Hamilton et al., "Default Mode and Task Positive Network Activity in Major Depressive Disorder: Implications for Adaptive and Maladaptive Rumination," *Biological Psychiatry* 70, no. 4 (2011): 327–33; Xueling Zhu et al., "Evidence of a Dissociation Pattern in Resting-State Default Mode Network Connectivity in First-Episode, Treatment-Naive Major Depression Patients," *Biological Psychiatry* 71, no. 7 (2012): 611; Christoff et al., "Mind-Wandering as Spontaneous Thought;" Roger E. Beaty et al., "Brain Networks of the Imaginative Mind: Dynamic Functional Connectivity of Default and Cognitive Control Networks Relates to Openness to Experience," *Human Brain Mapping* 39, no. 2 (2018): 811–21; Matthew L. Dixon et al., "Interactions between the Default Network and Dorsal Attention Network Vary across Default Subsystems, Time, and Cognitive States," *Neuroimage* 147 (2017): 632–49.

11. Ibid.

12. Ibid.

13. Ibid.

14. Cherbuin et al., "Validated Alzheimer's Disease Risk Index."

15. Leaf, *The Perfect You*; Sterling C. Johnson et al., "Neural Correlates of Self-Reflection," *Brain* 125, no. 8 (2002): 1808–14; Jack Mezirow, "How Critical Reflection Triggers Transformative Learning," *Fostering Critical Reflection in Adulthood* 1 (1990): 20.

16. Carey K. Morewedge, Colleen Giblin, and Michael I. Norton, "The (Perceived) Meaning of Spontaneous Thoughts," *Journal of Experimental Psychology: General* 143, no. 4 (August 2014): 1742–54.

17. Leaf, *The Perfect You*.

18. Richard Moulding et al., "They Scare Because We Care: The Relationship between Obsessive Intrusive Thoughts and Appraisals and Control Strategies across 15 Cities," *Journal of Obsessive-Compulsive and Related Disorders* 3, no. 3 (March 2014): 280–91.

19. Ibid.

20. Robert Berezin, "Psychiatric Diagnosis Is a Fraud: The Destructive and Damaging Fiction of Biological Diseases," *Mad in America*, April 5, 2016, https://www.madinamerica.com/2016/04/psychiatric-diagnosis-is-a-fraud-the-destructive-and-damaging-fiction-of-biological-diseases/.

21. William H. Davies, "Leisure Poem," *The Collected Poems of William H. Davies* (New York: A. A. Knopf, 1927), 18.

22. "Is Cell Phone Radiation Safe?" ProCon.org, https://cellphones.procon.org; "How Much Time Do People Spend on Their Mobile Phones in 2017?" *Hacker-Noon*, https://hackernoon.com/how-much-time-do-people-spend-on-their-mobile-phones-in-2017-e5f90a0b10a6; Stephanie Fanelli and Brian Wansink, "Surfing the Web While Fishing for Food: A Pilot Study Examining Cell Phone Use During Mealtime," *The FASEB Journal* 31, no. 1, supplement (2017), http://www.fasebj.org/doi/abs/10.1096/fasebj.31.1_supplement.957.35.

Chapter 3 The Controlled Thinking Mindset

1. John Sarno, *The Divided Mind: The Epidemic of Mindbody Disorders* (New York: Harper, 2006): 115.

2. Leaf, *Switch On Your Brain*; Leaf, *Think and Eat Yourself Smart*; Leaf, "21-Day Brain Detox."

3. Ibid.

4. Ibid.

5. Ibid.

6. Leaf, Uys, and Louw, "An Alternative Non-Traditional Approach to Learning;" Leaf, Uys, and Louw, "The Development of a Model for Geodesic Learning;" Leaf, Uys, and Louw, "The Mind Mapping Approach (MMA);" Leaf, Uys, and Louw, "Mind Mapping as a Therapeutic Intervention Technique;" Leaf, Uys, and Louw, "Mind Mapping as a Therapeutic Technique"; Leaf, Uys, and Louw, "Mind Mapping: A Therapeutic Technique for Closed Head Injury;" Leaf, Uys, and Louw, "The Move from Institution Based Rehabilitation (IBR) to Community Based Rehabilitation," *Therapy Africa* 1 (August 1997): 4.

7. Jason S. Moser et al., "Third-Person Self-Talk Facilitates Emotion Regulation without Engaging Cognitive Control: Converging Evidence from ERP and fMRI," *Scientific Reports* 7, no. 1 (2017): 4519.

8. Sonia J. Lupien et al., "Effects of Stress throughout the Lifespan on the Brain, Behaviour and Cognition," *Nature Reviews Neuroscience* 10, no. 6 (2009): 434–45.

9. Marian Cleeves Diamond, *Enriching Heredity: The Impact of the Environment on the Anatomy of the Brain* (New York: Free Press, 1988), David A. Sousa, *How the Brain Learns* (Newbury Park, CA: Corwin Press, 2016); Roberto Colom et al., "Brain Structural Changes following Adaptive Cognitive Training Assessed by Tensor-Based Morphometry (TBM)," *Neuropsychologia* 91 (2016): 77–85; Kirk I. Erickson, "Evidence for Structural Plasticity in Humans: Comment on Thomas and Baker (2012)," *NeuroImage* 73 (2013): 237–38; S. Katherine Nelson-Coffey et al., "Kindness in the Blood: A Randomized Controlled Trial of the Gene-Regulatory Impact of Prosocial Behavior," *Psychoneuroendocrinology* 81 (2017): 8–13; Kathi Norman, "Forgiveness: How it Manifests in Our Health, Well-being, and Longevity," *Master of Applied Positive Psychology (MAPP) Capstone Projects* 122, University of Pennsylvania (August 2017); http://repository.upenn.edu/mapp_capstone/122; Xueyi Shen et al., "Subcortical Volume and White Matter Integrity Abnormalities in Major Depressive Disorder: Findings from UK Biobank Imaging Data," *bioR xiv* (2017): 070912; Richard Restak, *The New Brain: How the Modern Age Is Rewiring Your Mind* (New York: Rodale, 2004); Daniel Goleman and Richard J. Davidson, *Altered Traits: Science Reveals How Meditation Changes Your Mind, Brain, and Body* (New York: Penguin, 2017); Conrad Wiegand, Andreas Savelsbergh, and Peter Heusser, "MicroRNAs in Psychological Stress Reactions and Their Use as Stress-Associated Biomarkers, Especially in Human Saliva," *Biomedicine Hub* 2, no. 3 (2017): 4; Miriam A. Schiele and Katharina Domschke, "Epigenetics at the Crossroads between Genes, Environment and Resilience in Anxiety Disorders," *Genes, Brain and Behavior* (September 2017).

10. John De Mado, "The Cognitive Benefits of Bilingualism/Biliteracy," *JDMLS*, accessed January 24, 2018, http://www.demado-seminars.com/archive/the_cognitive _benefits_of_bilingualism_biliteracy.htm; Diamond, *Enriching Heredity*; Graham W. Knott et al., "Formation of Dendritic Spines with GABAergic Synapses Induced by Whisker Stimulation in Adult Mice," *Neuron* 34, no. 2 (2002): 265–73; Maya Frankfurt and Victoria Luine, "The Evolving Role of Dendritic Spines and Memory: Interaction(s) with Estradiol," *Hormones and Behavior* 74 (2015): 28–36; Maria-Angeles Arevalo

et al., "Signaling Mechanisms Mediating the Regulation of Synaptic Plasticity and Memory by Estradiol," *Hormones and Behavior* 74 (2015): 19–27; Carl Fulwiler et al., "Mindfulness-Based Interventions for Weight Loss and CVD Risk Management," *Current Cardiovascular Risk Reports* 9, no. 10 (2015): 46; David Muehsam et al., "The Embodied Mind: a Review on Functional Genomic and Neurological Correlates of Mind-Body Therapies," *Neuroscience & Biobehavioral Reviews* 73 (2017): 165–81.

11. Leaf, "The Mind Mapping Approach."

12. Leaf, "The Mind Mapping Approach;" Leaf, "The Development of a Model for Geodesic Learning."

13. Ludwig H. Heydenreich, "Leonardo da Vinci, Architect of Francis I," *The Burlington Magazine* 94, no. 595 (1952): 277–85.

Chapter 4 The Words Mindset

1. Leaf, *Switch On Your Brain*; Leaf, *Think and Eat Yourself Smart*; Leaf, *The Perfect You*; Muehsam et al., "The Embodied Mind."

2. Diane Arathuzik, "Effects of Cognitive-Behavioral Strategies on Pain in Cancer Patients," *Cancer Nursing* 17, no. 3 (1994): 207–14; Robyn Lewis Brown, Mairead Eastin Moloney, and Gabriele Ciciurkaite, "People with Physical Disabilities, Work, and Well-being: The Importance of Autonomous and Creative Work," *Factors in Studying Employment for Persons with Disability: How the Picture Can Change* (Bingley, UK: Emerald Publishing Limited, 2017), 205–24; Joseph A. Schenk, "The Mobius Strip of Total Health: Manipulation of Thinking Prior to Exercise Activity," university honors program thesis, Georgia Southern University (2017); Tracey Anderson Askew, "The Power of Words!" *Australian Midwifery News* 17, no. 2 (2017): 26; Seth Peterson, "The Power of Words: James 3:1–12," graduate oral presentation, Liberty University, April 13, 2017, http://digitalcommons.liberty.edu/cgi/viewcontent.cgi?article=1097 &context=research_symp; Matthew Lieberman et al., "Putting Feelings Into Words," *Psychological Science* 18, no. 5 (May 2007): 421–28; Stuart Wolpert, "Putting Feelings Into Words Produces Therapeutic Effects in the Brain; UCLA Neuroimaging Study Supports Ancient Buddhist Teachings," *UCLA Newsroom* (June 21, 2007).

3. Lieberman et al., "Putting Feelings into Words;" Eric B. Loucks et al., "Positive Associations of Dispositional Mindfulness with Cardiovascular Health: The New England Family Study," *International Journal of Behavioral Medicine* 22, no. 4 (2015): 540–50; Muehsam et al., "The Embodied Mind."

Chapter 5 The Controlled Emotions Mindset

1. Muehsam et al., "The Embodied Mind;" Lieberman et al., "Putting Feelings Into Words;" Candace B. Pert, *Molecules of Emotion: Why You Feel the Way You Feel* (New York: Simon and Schuster, 1997); Margaret Wheatley, *Leadership and the New Science: Discovering Order in a Chaotic World* (San Francisco: Berrett-Koehler, 2006); Edmund T. Rolls, "On the Brain and Emotion," *Behavioral and Brain Sciences* 23, no. 2 (2000): 219–28.

2. Lisa Feldman Barrett, "You Aren't at the Mercy of Your Emotions—Your Brain Creates Them," TED talk, recorded December 2017 at TED@IBM, 18:29, https://www.ted.com/talks/lisa_feldman_barrett_you_aren_t_at_the_mercy_of_your_emotions_your_brain_creates_them.

3. Caroline Leaf, *Who Switched Off My Brain: Controlling Toxic Thoughts and Emotions* (Nashville: Thomas Nelson, 2009); Luiz Pessoa, "A Network Model of the Emotional Brain," *Trends in Cognitive Sciences* 21, no. 5 (May 2017): 357–71; Sophia Suk Mun Law, "Colour My Growth: A Study of Art as a Language for Victims of Family Violence," *Hong Kong Association of Art Therapists Newsletter* 25 (February 2017), http://commons.ln.edu.hk/sw_master/5277/; Heather Bacon, "Book Review: Jonathan Willows, Moving on after Childhood Sexual Abuse, Understanding the Effects and Preparing for Therapy," *Clinical Child Psychology and Psychiatry* 15, no. 1 (2010): 141–42.

Chapter 6 The Forgiveness Mindset

1. Saima Noreen, Raynette N. Bierman, and Malcolm D. MacLeod, "Forgiving You Is Hard, but Forgetting Seems Easy: Can Forgiveness Facilitate Forgetting?" *Psychological Science* 25, no. 7 (2014): 1295–302.

2. Nathaniel G. Wade et al., "Efficacy of Psychotherapeutic Interventions to Promote Forgiveness: A Meta-Analysis," *Forgiveness Therapy* (2014): 154; Don E. Davis et al., "Research on Religion/Spirituality and Forgiveness: A Meta-Analytic Review," *Psychology of Religion and Spirituality* 5, no. 4 (2013): 233; Robert D. Enright, *The Forgiving Life: A Pathway to Overcoming Resentment and Creating a Legacy of Love* (York, PA: Maple-Vail Books, 2012); Brandon J. Griffin et al., "Self-Directed Intervention to Promote Self-Forgiveness," *Handbook of the Psychology of Self-Forgiveness* (Berlin: Springer, 2017), 207–18.

3. Indrajeet Patil et al., "Neuroanatomical Correlates of Forgiving Unintentional Harms," *Scientific Reports* 7 (2017); Noreen, Bierman, and MacLeod, "Forgiving You Is Hard;" Stephanie Lichtenfeld et al., "Forgive and Forget: Differences between Decisional and Emotional Forgiveness," *PLoS One* 10, no. 5 (2015): e0125561; Whitney K. Jeter and Laura A. Brannon, "Increasing Awareness of Potentially Helpful Motivations and Techniques for Forgiveness," *Counseling and Values* 60, no. 2 (2015): 186–200; C. Fred Alford, "Forgiveness and Transitional Experience," *D. W. Winnicott and Political Theory* (New York: Palgrave Macmillan, 2017), 185–201.

4. Mayo Clinic, "Learning to Forgive May Improve Well-Being," *ScienceDaily*, January 4, 2008, https://www.sciencedaily.com/releases/2008/01/080104122807.htm.

5. Ibid.

Chapter 7 The Happiness Mindset

1. Greater Good Science Center at UC Berkeley, "Emiliana R. Simon-Thomas: Profile," *Greater Good Magazine*, accessed January 24, 2018, https://greatergood .berkeley.edu/profile/emiliana_simon_thomas; Dacher Keltner, *Born to Be Good: The Science of a Meaningful Life* (New York: WW Norton, 2009).

2. Kent C. Berridge, "'Liking' and 'Wanting' Food Rewards: Brain Substrates and Roles in Eating Disorders," *Physiology & Behavior* 97, no. 5 (2009): 537–50; W. Bradford Littlejohn, "Addicted to Novelty: The Vice of Curiosity in a Digital Age," *Journal of the Society of Christian Ethics* 37, no. 1 (2017): 179–96; Daniel Pedro Cardinali, "Fourth Level: The Limbic System," *Autonomic Nervous System* (Berlin: Springer, 2018), 245–85.

3. Achor, *Happiness Advantage*.

4. Sonja Lyubomirsky, Laura King, and Ed Diener, "The Benefits of Frequent Positive Affect: Does Happiness Lead to Success?" *PubMed* (2005): 803, doi: 10.1037 /0033-2909.131.6.803.

5. Achor, *Happiness Advantage*; Crum, Salovey, and Achor, "Rethinking Stress;" John B. Izzo, *The Five Thieves of Happiness* (Oakland, CA: Berrett-Koehler, 2017); L. Parker Schiffer and Tomi-Ann Roberts, "The Paradox of Happiness: Why Are We Not Doing What We Know Makes Us Happy?" *The Journal of Positive Psychology* (January 2017): 1–8.

6. Ibid.

7. Ibid.

8. Ellen Beth Levitt, "University of Maryland School of Medicine Study Shows Laughter Helps Blood Vessels Function Better," University of Maryland Medical Center, March 9, 2009 [cited October 25, 2011]; Julia Wilkins and Amy Janel Eisenbraun, "Humor Theories and the Physiological Benefits of Laughter," *Holistic Nursing Practice* 23, no. 6 (2009): 349–54; Sala Horowitz, "Effect of Positive Emotions on Health: Hope and Humor," *Alternative and Complimentary Therapies* 15, no. 4 (2009): 196–202; Norman Cousins, "Anatomy of an Illness (as Perceived by the Patient)," *Nutrition Today* 12, no. 3 (1977): 22–28; Norman Cousins, "Therapeutic Value of Laughter," *Integrative Psychiatry* (1985); Norman Cousins, "Proving the Power of Laughter," *Psychology Today* 23, no. 10 (1989): 22–25; Brandon M. Savage et al., "Humor, Laughter, Learning, and Health! A Brief Review," *Advances in Physiology Education* 41, no. 3 (2017): 341–47; Allen B. Weisse, "Humor in Medicine: Can Laughter Help in Healing?" *Proceedings (Baylor University Medical Center)* 30, no. 3 (2017): 378; Mohamed H. Noureldein and Assaad A. Eid, "Homeostatic Effect of Laughter on Diabetic Cardiovascular Complications: The Myth Turned to Fact," *Diabetes Research and Clinical Practice* 135 (January 2018): 111–19; Elisabeth Ritter, "Laughing to Heal and Renew: Implementation of Humor in Dance/Movement Therapy," graduate thesis, Sarah Lawrence College (May 2017); Frank Rodden, "The Neurology and Psychiatry of Humor, Smiling and Laughter: A Tribute to Paul McGhee, Part I, Introduction and Clinical Studies," *Humor* (January 2017); Lee S. Berk et al., "Neuroendocrine and Stress Hormone Changes During Mirthful Laughter," *The American Journal of the Medical Sciences* 298, no. 6 (1989): 390–96.

9. Ibid.

10. Ibid.

11. Ibid.

12. Robert R. Provine, "Laughter as an Approach to Vocal Evolution: The Bipedal Theory," *Psychonomic Bulletin & Review* 24, no. 1 (2017): 238–44.

13. Ruby T. Nadler, Rahel Rabi, and John Paul Minda, "Better Mood and Better Performance: Learning Rule-Described Categories Is Enhanced by Positive Mood," *Psychological Science* 21, no. 12 (2010): 1770–76.

Chapter 8 The Time Mindset

1. Jamil P. Bhanji and Mauricio R. Delgado, "Perceived Control Influences Neural Responses to Setbacks and Promotes Persistence," *Neuron* 83, no. 6 (2014): 1369–75; Lauren A. Leotti, Catherine Cho, and Mauricio R. Delgado, "The Neural Basis Underlying the Experience of Control in the Human Brain," *The Sense of*

Agency, edited by Patrick Haggard and Baruch Eitam (Oxford Scholarship Online, 2015): 145.

2. Phillippa Lally et al., "How Are Habits Formed: Modelling Habit Formation in the Real World," *European Journal of Social Psychology* 40, no. 6 (2010): 998–1009; Phillippa Lally and Benjamin Gardner, "Promoting Habit Formation," *Health Psychology Review* 7, supplement 1 (2013): S137–58; Sheina Orbell and Bas Verplanken, "The Automatic Component of Habit in Health Behavior: Habit as Cue-Contingent Automaticity," *Health Psychology* 29, no. 4 (2010): 374; Phillippa Lally, Jane Wardle, and Benjamin Gardner, "Experiences of Habit Formation: A Qualitative Study," *Psychology, Health & Medicine* 16, no. 4 (2011): 484–89.

Chapter 9 The Possible Mindset

1. Neil Garrett and Tali Sharot, "Optimistic Update Bias Holds Firm: Three Tests of Robustness Following Shah et al.," *Consciousness and Cognition* 50 (2017): 12–22; Sharot et al., "Neural Mechanisms Mediating Optimism Bias;" Sharot, "The Optimism Bias;" Sharot, *The Optimism Bias*; Tali Sharot et al., "How Dopamine Enhances an Optimism Bias in Humans," *Current Biology* 22, no. 16 (2012): 1477–81.

2. Rutgers School of Arts and Sciences, *The Edisonian* 9 (Fall 2012), http.//edison .rutgers.edu/newsletter9.html.

3. Achor, *Happiness Advantage*.

Chapter 10 The Gratitude Mindset

1. Prathik Kini et al., "The Effects of Gratitude Expression on Neural Activity," *NeuroImage* 128 (2016): 1–10, https://www.ncbi.nlm.nih.gov/pubmed/26746580; Sungh-yon Kyeong et al., "Effects of Gratitude Meditation on Neural Network Functional Connectivity and Brain-Heart Coupling," *Scientific Reports* 7, no. 1 (2017): 5058

2. Kini et al., "Effects of Gratitude Expression."

3. Kini et al., "Effects of Gratitude Expression;" Robert A. Emmons, *Thanks! How the New Science of Gratitude Can Make You Happier* (New York: Houghton Mifflin Harcourt, 2007); Philip C. Watkins, Dean L. Grimm, and Russell Kolts, "Counting Your Blessings: Positive Memories among Grateful Persons," *Current Psychology* 23, no. 1 (2004): 52–67; Sonja Lyubomirsky, *The How of Happiness: A Scientific Approach to Getting the Life You Want* (New York: Penguin, 2008); Anna Alkozei, Ryan Smith, and William D. S. Killgore, "Gratitude and Subjective Wellbeing: A Proposal of Two Causal Frameworks," *Journal of Happiness Studies* (2017): 1–24; Alex M. Wood et al., "The Role of Gratitude in the Development of Social Support, Stress, and Depression: Two Longitudinal Studies," *Journal of Research in Personality* 42, no. 4 (2008): 854–71; Stephen M. Yoshimura and Kassandra Berzins, "Grateful Experiences and Expressions: The Role of Gratitude Expressions in the Link between Gratitude Experiences and Well-Being," *Review of Communication* 17, no. 2 (2017): 106–18.

4. Alexis Madrigal, "Scanning Dead Salmon in FMRI Machine Highlights Risk of Red Herrings," *Wired*, September 19, 2009, https://www.wired.com/2009/09/fm risalmon; Brian Resnick, "There's a Lot of Junk FMRI Research Out There: Here's What Top Neuroscientists Want You to Know," *Vox*, September 9, 2016, http://www .vox.com/2016/9/8/1289784?fmri-studies-explained.

5. Robert A. Emmons and Michael E. McCullough, eds., *The Psychology of Gratitude* (London: Oxford University Press, 2004), 232.

6. Toshimasa Sone et al., "Sense of Life Worth Living (Ikigai) and Mortality in Japan: Ohsaki Study," *Psychosomatic Medicine* 70, no. 6 (2008): 709–15.

7. Willie Nelson and Turk Pipkin, *The Tao of Willie: A Guide to the Happiness in Your Heart* (New York: Gotham, 2007), xii.

Chapter 11 The Community Mindset

1. Roger Walsh, "Lifestyle and Mental Health," *American Psychologist* 66, no. 7 (2011): 579; Bruce E. Wampold and Zac E. Imel, *The Great Psychotherapy Debate: The Evidence for What Makes Psychotherapy Work* (London: Routledge, 2015); Roger Walsh, "Integral Service, Part 2: Integral Discipline, Karma Yoga, and Sacred Service," *Journal of Integral Theory and Practice* 9, no. 1 (2014): 132; Kellsey D. Calhoon, "Getting Off the Couch: Psychotherapists Who Have Incorporated Therapeutic Lifestyle Changes into Their Practice," graduate thesis, University of Alberta (2014); Glenn Hutchinson, "Mental Health 101: How To Improve Your Mental Health Without Going to Therapy," *Glenn Hutchinson, Ph.D.*, accessed January 25, 2018, http://glennhutchinson.net/How-To-Improve-Your-Mental-Health.html; Amrita Yadava, Deepti Hooda, and NovRattan Sharma, "Maintaining and Improving Health through Lifestyle Choices," *Biopsychosocial Issues in Positive Health*, edited by Amrita Yadava, Deepti Hooda, and NovRattan Sharma (New Delhi, India: Global Vision, 2012).

2. D. B. López Lluch and L. Noguera Artiaga, "The Sense of Touch," *Sensory and Aroma Marketing* (Wageningen, Netherlands: Wageningen Academic Publishers, 2017), 472–88; Jenn Gonya et al., "Investigating Skin-to-Skin Care Patterns with Extremely Preterm Infants in the NICU and Their Effect on Early Cognitive and Communication Performance: A Retrospective Cohort Study," *BMJ open* 7, no. 3 (2017): e012985; Dorothy Vittner et al., "Increase in Oxytocin from Skin-to-Skin Contact Enhances Development of Parent-Infant Relationship," *Biological Research for Nursing* 20, no. 1 (October 2017): 54–62; Alessandro Sale, "A Systematic Look at Environmental Modulation and Its Impact in Brain Development," *Trends in Neurosciences* 41, no. 1 (January 2018): 4–17; Anne C. Rovers et al., "Effectiveness of Skin-to-Skin Contact versus Care-as-Usual in Mothers and Their Full-Term Infants: Study Protocol for a Parallel-Group Randomized Controlled Trial," *BMC Pediatrics* 17, no. 1 (2017): 154; Joan L. Luby et al., "Association between Early Life Adversity and Risk for Poor Emotional and Physical Health in Adolescence: A Putative Mechanistic Neurodevelopmental Pathway," *JAMA Pediatrics* 171, no. 12 (2017): 1168–75.

3. Zenobia Morrill, "Loneliness as Lethal: Researchers Name Social Isolation a 'Public Health Threat,'" *Mad in America*, September 1, 2017, https://www.madinamerica.com/2017/09/loneliness-lethal-researchers-name-social-isolation-public-health-threat/; Holt-Lunstad et al., "Loneliness and Social Isolation as Risk Factors for Mortality;" Stephanie Cacioppo et al., "Loneliness: Clinical Import and Interventions," *Perspectives on Psychological Science* 10, no. 2 (2015): 238–49; Riitta Hari et al., "Centrality of Social Interaction in Human Brain Function," *Neuron* 88, no. 1 (2015): 181–93; Nicole K. Valtorta et al., "Loneliness and Social Isolation as Risk Factors for Coronary Heart Disease and Stroke: Systematic Review and Meta-Analysis of Longitudinal Observational Studies," *Heart* 102, no. 13 (2016): 1009–16.

4. Holt-Lunstad et al., "Loneliness and Social Isolation as Risk Factors for Mortality;" Sebastian Mann, "Loneliness 'Kills More People than Obesity,'" *Evening Standard*, August 7, 2017, https://www.standard.co.uk/news/health/loneliness-kills-more-people -than-obesity-a3605786.html.

5. Ibid.

6. Ibid.

7. American Psychological Association, "How Do Close Relationships Lead to Longer Life?" *ScienceDaily*, September 7, 2017, www.sciencedaily.com/releases/2017 /09/170907093638.htm.

8. As quoted in Hooseo B. Park, *The Eight Answers for Happiness* (Bloomington, IN: Xlibris, 2014), 105.

9. Holt-Lunstad et al., "Loneliness and Social Isolation as Risk Factors for Mortality."

10. Ibid.

11. To learn more, visit www.wholemindproject.com.

12. Dixon Chibanda et al., "Effect of a Primary Care–Based Psychological Intervention on Symptoms of Common Mental Disorders in Zimbabwe: A Randomized Clinical Trial," *JAMA* 316, no. 24 (2016): 2618–26.

Chapter 12 The Support Mindset

1. Holt-Lunstad et al., "Loneliness and Social Isolation as Risk Factors for Mortality."

2. Brooke C. Feeney et al., "Predicting the Pursuit and Support of Challenging Life Opportunities," *Personality and Social Psychology Bulletin* 43, no. 8 (August 2017): 1171–87.

3. Frank J. Infurna and Suniya S. Luthar, "Resilience to Major Life Stressors Is Not as Common as Thought," *Perspectives on Psychological Science* 11, no. 2 (2016): 175–94; Suzanne Degges-White and Christine Borzumato-Gainey, *Friends Forever: How Girls and Women Forge Lasting Relationships* (London: Rowman & Littlefield, 2011); Suzanne Degges-White, *Sisters and Brothers for Life: Making Sense of Sibling Relationships in Adulthood* (London: Rowman & Littlefield, 2017); Christine Borzumato-Gainey, Suzanne Degges-White, and Carrie V. Smith, "Romantic Relationships: From Wrestling to Romance," *Counseling Boys and Young Men*, edited by Suzanne Degges-White and Bonnie Colon (Berlin: Springer, 2012), 135.

4. Holt-Lunstad et al., "Loneliness and Social Isolation as Risk Factors for Mortality."

5. M. J. Poulin et al., "Giving to Others and the Association between Stress and Mortality," *Am J Public Health* 103, no. 9 (September 2013): 1649–55; E. B. Raposa, H. B. Laws, and E. B. Ansell, "Prosocial Behavior Mitigates the Negative Effects of Stress in Everyday Life," *Clinical Psychological Science* 4, no. 4 (2016): 691–98.

6. Shawn Achor, "Positive Intelligence," *Harvard Business Review* 90, no. 1 (2012): 100–102; Achor, *Happiness Advantage*.

7. Ibid.

Chapter 13 The Healthy Stress Mindset

1. Jamieson, Mendes, and Nock, "Improving Acute Stress Responses;" Crum, Salovey, and Achor, "Rethinking Stress;" Anne Casper, Sabine Sonnentag, and Stephanie Tremmel, "Mindset Matters: the Role of Employees' Stress Mindset for Day-Specific Reactions to Workload Anticipation," *European Journal of Work and Organizational*

Psychology 26, no. 6 (2017): 1–13; M. J. Poulin et al., "Giving to Others and the Association between Stress and Mortality;" E. B. Raposa, H. B. Laws, and E. B. Ansell, "Prosocial Behavior Mitigates the Negative Effects of Stress in Everyday Life;" Jeremy P. Jamieson et al., "Capitalizing on Appraisal Processes to Improve Affective Responses to Social Stress," *Emotion Review* (2017), doi:1754073917693085; Beltzer et al., "Rethinking Butterflies;" Marcie A. LePine et al., "Turning Their Pain to Gain: Charismatic Leader Influence on Follower Stress Appraisal and Job Performance," *Academy of Management Journal* 59, no. 3 (2016): 1036–59; Angela L. Duckworth, Tamar Szabó Gendler, and James J. Gross, "Self-Control in School-Age Children," *Educational Psychologist* 49, no. 3 (2014): 199–217; Jamieson et al., "Turning the Knots in Your Stomach into Bows;" Nancy L. Sin et al., "Linking Daily Stress Processes and Laboratory-Based Heart Rate Variability in a National Sample of Midlife and Older Adults," *Psychosomatic Medicine* 78, no. 5 (2016): 573–82.

2. Ibid.
3. Ibid.
4. Ibid.
5. Ibid.
6. Crum, Salovey, and Achor, "Rethinking Stress."

Chapter 14 The Expectancy Mindset

1. Crum and Langer, "Mind-Set Matters."
2. Ibid.
3. Jon D. Levine, Newton C. Gordon, and Howard L. Fields, "The Mechanism of Placebo Analgesia," *The Lancet* 312, no. 8091 (1978): 654–57.
4. Martina Amanzio and Fabrizio Benedetti, "Neuropharmacological Dissection of Placebo Analgesia: Expectation-Activated Opioid Systems versus Conditioning-Activated Specific Subsystems," *Journal of Neuroscience* 19, no. 1 (1999): 484–94.
5. Jo Marchant, "Placebos: Honest Fakery," *Nature* 535, no. 7611 (2016): S14–15, http://www.nature.com/nature/journal/v535/n7611_supp/full/535S14a.html#ref3.
6. Marchant, "Placebos;" Tor D. Wager and Lauren Y. Atlas, "The Neuroscience of Placebo Effects: Connecting Context, Learning and Health," *Nature Reviews Neuroscience* 16, no. 7 (2015): 403–18; Fadel Zeidan et al., "Mindfulness Meditation-Based Pain Relief Employs Different Neural Mechanisms than Placebo and Sham Mindfulness Meditation-Induced Analgesia," *Journal of Neuroscience* 35, no. 46 (2015): 15307–25; Cláudia Carvalho et al., "Open-Label Placebo Treatment in Chronic Low Back Pain: A Randomized Controlled Trial," *Pain* 157, no. 12 (2016): 2766; Damien G. Finniss et al., "Biological, Clinical, and Ethical Advances of Placebo Effects," *The Lancet* 375, no. 9715 (2010): 686–95.
7. Ibid.
8. Finniss et al., "Biological, Clinical, and Ethical Advances of Placebo Effects."
9. Herbert Spiegel, "Nocebo: the Power of Suggestibility," *Preventive Medicine* 26, no. 5 (1997): 616–21; Guy H. Montgomery and Irving Kirsch, "Classical Conditioning and the Placebo Effect," *Pain* 72, no. 1 (1997): 107–13; Steve Stewart-Williams and John Podd, "The Placebo Effect: Dissolving the Expectancy versus Conditioning Debate," *Psychological Bulletin* 130, no. 2 (2004): 324.

10. Fabrizio Benedetti, Elisa Carlino, and Antonella Pollo, "How Placebos Change the Patient's Brain," *Neuropsychopharmacology* 36, no. 1 (2011): 339–54.

11. Fabrizio Benedetti et al., "When Words Are Painful: Unraveling the Mechanisms of the Nocebo Effect," *Neuroscience* 147, no. 2 (2007): 260–71.

12. Benedetti, Carlino, and Pollo, "How Placebos Change the Patient's Brain."

Chapter 15 The Willpower Mindset

1. Roland Bénabou and Jean Tirole, "Willpower and Personal Rules," *Journal of Political Economy* 112, no. 4 (2004): 848–86; Vaughan Michell and Jasmine Tehrani, "Clinical Pathways and the Human Factor: Approaches to Control and Reduction of Human Error Risk," *Impact of Medical Errors and Malpractice on Health Economics, Quality, and Patient Safety*, edited by Marina Riga (Hershey, PA: Medical Information Science Reference, 2017); Martin G. Kocher et al., "Strong, Bold, and Kind: Self-Control and Cooperation in Social Dilemmas," *Experimental Economics* 20, no. 1 (2017): 44–69; Carol Dweck, *Mindset: Changing the Way You Think to Fulfill Your Potential* (London: Hachette UK, 2017); Urshila Sriram et al., "Support and Sabotage: A Qualitative Study of Social Influences on Health Behaviors among Rural Adults," *The Journal of Rural Health* 34, no. 1 (2018): 88–97.

2. Ibid.

3. Peter J. Rogers, "A Healthy Body, a Healthy Mind: Long-Term Impact of Diet on Mood and Cognitive Function," *Proceedings of the Nutrition Society* 60, no. 1 (2001): 135–43; Lawrence Friedman, "How the Mind-Gut Connection Affects Your Health: The 'Second Brain' in Your Stomach Can Cause or Relieve Illness and Stress. Here's How It Works," *Next Avenue*, June 19, 2013, http://www.nextavenue.org /how-mind-gut-connection-affects-your-health/; Ruth Anne Luna and Jane A. Foster, "Gut Brain Axis: Diet Microbiota Interactions and Implications for Modulation of Anxiety and Depression," *Current Opinion in Biotechnology* 32 (April 2015): 35–41; Philip C. Keightley, Natasha A. Koloski, and Nicholas J. Talley, "Pathways in Gut-Brain Communication: Evidence for Distinct Gut-to-Brain and Brain-to-Gut Syndromes," *Australian and New Zealand Journal of Psychiatry* 49, no. 3 (2015): 207–14; Leaf, *Think and Eat Yourself Smart*.

Chapter 16 The Spiritual Mindset

1. Dan Buettner, *The Blue Zones: 9 Lessons for Living Longer from the People Who've Lived the Longest* (Des Moines, IA: National Geographic Books, 2012).

2. Christina M. Puchalski, "The Role of Spirituality in Health Care," *Proceedings (Baylor University Medical Center)* 14, no. 4 (2001): 352; Gowri Anandarajah and Ellen Hight, "Spirituality and Medical Practice," *American Family Physician* 63, no. 1 (2001): 81–88; Rush University Medical Center, "Belief in a Caring God Improves Response to Medical Treatment for Depression, Study Finds," *ScienceDaily*, February 24, 2010, www.sciencedaily.com/releases/2010/02/100223132021.htm; David H. Rosmarin et al., "A Test of Faith in God and Treatment: The Relationship of Belief in God to Psychiatric Treatment Outcomes," *Journal of Affective Disorders* 146, no. 3 (2013): 441–46; Bruno Paz Mosqueiro, Neusa Sica da Rocha, and Marcelo Pio de Almeida Fleck, "Intrinsic Religiosity, Resilience, Quality of Life, and Suicide Risk in Depressed Inpatients," *Journal of Affective Disorders* 179 (2015): 128–33; Anne-Marie

Snider and Samara McPhedran, "Religiosity, Spirituality, Mental Health, and Mental Health Treatment Outcomes in Australia: A Systematic Literature Review," *Mental Health, Religion & Culture* 17, no. 6 (2014): 568–81; Freda van der Walt and Jeremias J. de Klerk, "Measuring Spirituality in South Africa: Validation of Instruments Developed in the USA," *International Review of Psychiatry* 26, no. 3 (2014): 368–78; Loren L. Toussaint, Justin C. Marschall, and David R. Williams, "Prospective Associations between Religiousness/Spirituality and Depression and Mediating Effects of Forgiveness in a Nationally Representative Sample of United States Adults," *Depression Research and Treatment* 2012 (2012).

3. Ibid.

4. Alister E. McGrath, *Surprised by Meaning: Science, Faith, and How We Make Sense of Things* (Louisville: Westminster John Knox, 2011); Alister E. McGrath, *Science & Religion: A New Introduction* (West Sussex, UK: Wiley-Blackwell, 2010); Alister E. McGrath, *Why God Won't Go Away: Is the New Atheism Running on Empty?* (Nashville: Thomas Nelson, 2010); J. C. Polkinghorne, *Science and Religion in Quest of Truth* (New Haven, CT: Yale University Press, 2011); J. C. Polkinghorne, *Belief in God in an Age of Science* (New Haven, CT: Yale University Press, 1998); J. C. Polkinghorne, *One World: The Interaction of Science and Theology* (Philadelphia: Templeton Foundation Press, 2007); J. C. Polkinghorne and Nicholas Beale, *Questions of Truth: Fifty-One Responses to Questions about God, Science, and Belief* (Louisville: Westminster John Knox, 2009); John C. Lennox, *Seven Days That Divide the World: The Beginning According to Genesis and Science* (Grand Rapids: Zondervan, 2011); Amir D. Aczel, *Why Science Does Not Disprove God* (New York: William Morrow, 2014); Andrew B. Newberg, Eugene G. D'Aquili, and Vince Rause, *Why God Won't Go Away: Brain Science and the Biology of Belief* (New York: Ballantine, 2001); Alister E. McGrath, *Darwinism and the Divine: Evolutionary Thought and Natural Theology* (Oxford, UK: Wiley-Blackwell, 2011).

5. Hill, Edmonds, and Hampson, "A Purposeful Lifestyle Is a Healthful Lifestyle."

6. Patrick L. Hill and Nicholas A. Turiano, "Purpose in Life as a Predictor of Mortality across Adulthood," *Psychological Science* 25, no. 7 (2014): 1482–86.

7. Viktor Emil Frankl, *Man's Search for Meaning: An Introduction to Logotherapy from Death-Camp to Existentialism* (New York: Simon & Schuster, 1962).

Chapter 17 The Purpose of the Gift Profile

1. Binghamton University, "Researchers Can Identify You by Your Brain Waves with 100 Percent Accuracy," *ScienceDaily*, April 18, 2016, https://www.sciencedaily.com/releases/2016/04/160418120608.htm; Maria V. Ruiz-Blondet et al., "A Novel Method for Very High Accuracy Event-Related Potential Biometric Identification," *CEREBRE: IEEE Transactions on Information Forensics and Security* 11, no. 7 (2016): 1618; Weizmann Institute of Science, "Smell Fingerprints? Each Person May Have a Unique Sense of Smell," *ScienceDaily*, June 30, 2015, www.sciencedaily.com/releases/2015/06/150630100509.htm; Eric A. Franzosa et al., "Identifying Personal Microbiomes Using Metagenomic Codes," *Proceedings of the National Academy of Sciences* 112, no. 22 (2015): E2930–38; Glendon J. Parker et al., "Demonstration of Protein-Based Human Identification Using the Hair Shaft Proteome," *PloS One* 11, no. 9 (2016): e0160653.

2. Tim Spector, "Identically Different: Tim Spector at TEDxKingsCollegeLondon," YouTube video, 18:15, uploaded by TEDx Talks, May 23, 2013, https://youtu.be/1W5SeBYERNI; Jordana T. Bell and Tim D. Spector, "A Twin Approach to Unraveling Epigenetics," *Trends in Genetics* 27, no. 3 (2011): 116–25; Jordana T. Bell and Richard Saffery, "The Value of Twins in Epigenetic Epidemiology," *International Journal of Epidemiology* 41, no. 1 (2012): 140–50; Tim Spector, *Identically Different: Why We Can Change Our Genes* (New York: Overlook Press, 2014).

3. Athanasia D. Panopoulos et al., "Aberrant DNA Methylation in Human iPSCs Associates with MYC-Binding Motifs in a Clone-Specific Manner Independent of Genetics," *Cell Stem Cell* 20, no. 4 (2017): 505–17; Cosmas D. Arnold et al., "Genome-Wide Quantitative Enhancer Activity Maps Identified by STARR=Seq," *Science* 339, no. 6123 (March 1, 2013): 1074–77; L. I. Patrushev and T. F. Kovalenko, "Functions of Noncoding Sequences in Mammalian Genomes," *Biochemistry (Mosc.)* 79, no. 13 (December 2014): 1442–69; Manolis Kellis et al., "Defining Functional DNA Elements in the Human Genome," *Proc Natl Acad Sci USA* 111, no. 17 (April 29, 2014): 6131 38; Perla Kaliman et al., "Rapid Changes in Histone Deacetylases and Inflammatory Gene Expression in Expert Meditators," *Psychoneuroendocrinology* 40 (February 2014): 96–107.

4. Ibid.

5. Zsofia Nemoda and Moshe Szyf, "Epigenetic Alterations and Prenatal Maternal Depression," *Birth Defects Research* 109, no. 12 (2017): 888–97; Trygve Tollefsbol, ed., *Handbook of Epigenetics: The New Molecular and Medical Genetics* (New York: Elsevier/Academic Press, 2011); Bruce H. Lipton, *The Biology of Belief: Unleashing the Power of Consciousness, Matter, and Miracles* (Carlsbad, CA: Hay House, 2008); R. Restak, *Mysteries of the Mind* (Washington, DC: National Geographic, 2000); Moshe Szyf, "Epigenetics, DNA Methylation, and Chromatin Modifying Drugs," *Annual Review of Pharmacology and Toxicology* 49 (2009): 243–63.

6. B. H. Lipton, "Insight into Cellular Consciousness;" Marc Folcher et al., "Mind-Controlled Transgene Expression by a Wireless-Powered Optogenetic Designer Cell Implant," *Nature Communications* 5 (2014), doi:10.1038/ncomms6392; Shawn Wu, Lin Jiang, and J. Wang, "From Relaxation Response, Building Power for Health to an Advanced Self-Cultivation Practice: Genuine Well-Being," *Well-Being and Quality of Life—Medical Perspective*, edited by Mukadder Mollaoglu (London: InTech, 2017); Massachusetts General Hospital, "Relaxation Response Can Influence Expression Of Stress-Related Genes," *ScienceDaily*, July 3, 2008, www.sciencedaily.com/releases/2008/07/080701221501.htm; Bruce D. Perry, "Childhood Experience and the Expression of Genetic Potential: What Childhood Neglect Tells Us about Nature and Nurture," *Brain and Mind* 3, no. 1 (2002): 79–100; Susan C. South, Nayla R. Hamdi, and Robert F. Krueger, "Biometric Modeling of Gene-Environment Interplay: The Intersection of Theory and Method and Applications for Social Inequality," *Journal of Personality* 85, no. 1 (2017): 22–37; Gene E. Robinson, Russell D. Fernald, and David F. Clayton, "Genes and Social Behavior," *Science* 322, no. 5903 (2008): 896–900; Ivana Buric et al., "What Is the Molecular Signature of Mind–Body Interventions? A Systematic Review of Gene Expression Changes Induced by Meditation and Related Practices," *Frontiers in Immunology* 8 (2017): 670; Yi Seok Chang et al., "Stress-Inducible Gene Atf3 in the Noncancer Host Cells Contributes to Chemotherapy-Exacerbated Breast Cancer Metastasis," *Proceedings of the National Academy of Sciences* 114, no. 34 (2017):

E7159–68; Nicole D. Powell et al., "Social Stress Up-Regulates Inflammatory Gene Expression in the Leukocyte Transcriptome via β-Adrenergic Induction of Myelopoiesis," *Proceedings of the National Academy of Sciences* 110, no. 41 (2013): 16574–79; Ohio State University, "Effects of Chronic Stress Can Be Traced to Your Genes," *Science-Daily*, November 5, 2013, www.sciencedaily.com/releases/2013/11/131105171338.htm; Steven W. Cole et al., "Transcript Origin Analysis Identifies Antigen-Presenting Cells as Primary Targets of Socially Regulated Gene Expression in Leukocytes," *Proceedings of the National Academy of Sciences* 108, no. 7 (2011): 3080–85; Daniel B. McKim et al., "Neuroinflammatory Dynamics Underlie Memory Impairments after Repeated Social Defeat," *Journal of Neuroscience* 36, no. 9 (2016): 2590–604; Dweck, *Mindset: Changing the Way You Think to Fulfill Your Potential*; Carol S. Dweck, *Mindset: The New Psychology of Success* (New York: Random House, 2006).

7. Ibid.

8. Leaf, *Switch On Your Brain*; Leaf, *Think and Eat Yourself Smart*; Leaf, *The Perfect You*.

9. Ibid.

10. Ibid.

11. Leaf, *The Perfect You*.

12. Ibid.

13. Joanna Moncrieff, "Philosophy Part 3: Knowledge of Mental States and Behaviour—Insights from Heidegger and Others," Joannamoncrieff.com, October 9, 2017, https://joannamoncrieff.com/2017/10/09/philosophy-part-3-knowledge-of-mental-states-and-behaviour-insights-from-heidegger-and-others/.

14. Michael Pollan, *The Omnivore's Dilemma: A Natural History of Four Meals* (New York: Penguin, 2006).

15. David J. Chalmers, *The Conscious Mind: In Search of a Fundamental Theory* (London: Oxford University Press, 1996).

16. Sally Satel and Scott O. Lilienfeld, *Brainwashed: The Seductive Appeal of Mindless Neuroscience* (New York: Basic Books, 2015); J. Kulnych, "Psychiatric Neuroimaging Evidence: A High-Tech Crystal Ball?" *Stanford Law Review* 49 (1997): 1249–70; E. Monterosso et al., "Explaining away Responsibility: Effects of Scientific Explanations on Perceived Culpability," *Ethics and Behavior* 15, no. 2 (2005): 139–53.

17. Brian Resnick, "There's a Lot of Junk FMRI Research out There;" A. Eklund et al., "Cluster Failure: Why FMRI Inferences for Spatial Extent Have Inflated False-Positive Rates," *Proceedings of the National Academy of Sciences* 113, no. 28 (2016): 7900–05.

18. Ibid.

19. Madrigal, "Scanning Dead Salmon."

20. Ibid.

21. Robert M. G. Reinhart, "Disruption and Rescue of Interareal Theta Phase Coupling and Adaptive Behavior," *Proceedings of the National Academy of Sciences* (2017): 11542–47; Boston University, "'Turbo Charge' for Your Brain? Sychronizing Specific Brain Occilations Enhances Executive Function," *ScienceDaily*, October 9, 2017, https://www.sciencedaily.com/releases/2017/10/171009154941.htm.

22. Stapp, "Quantum Interactive-Dualism."

23. Henry P. Stapp, *Mind, Matter and Quantum Mechanics* (Berlin: Springer, 2009), Kindle ed.

24. Leaf, "The Mind Mapping Approach: A Model and Framework for Geodesic Learning."
25. Henry Stapp, "Minds and Values in the Quantum Universe," *Information and the Nature of Reality from Physics to Metaphysics*, ed. P. C. W. Davies and Niels Henrik Gregersen (Cambridge, UK: Cambridge University Press, 2014), 157.
26. Roger Penrose, *Fashion, Faith, and Fantasy in the New Physics of the Universe* (Princeton, NJ: Princeton University Press, 2016).
27. Roger Penrose, *The Emperor's New Mind: Concerning Computers, Minds, and the Laws of Physics* (London: Oxford Paperbacks, 1999).
28. Ibid., 423.
29. Ibid.
30. Dr. Seuss, *Happy Birthday to You* (New York: Random House, 1959).
31. Leaf, "The Mind Mapping Approach: A Model and Framework for Geodesic Learning."
32. Stephen J. DeArmond, Madeline M. Fusco, and Maynard M. Dewey, *Structure of the Human Brain: A Photographic Atlas* (New York: Oxford University Press, 1989).
33. J. Fodor, *The Modularity of Mind* (Cambridge, MA: MIT/Bradford, 1989); Henry Markram, "The Blue Brain Project," *Nature Reviews Neuroscience* 7, no. 2 (2006): 153–60; Henry Markram, "The Human Brain Project," *Scientific American* 306, no. 6 (2012): 50–55; Jeffrey M. Schwartz, Henry P. Stapp, and Mario Beauregard, "Quantum Physics in Neuroscience and Psychology: A Neurophysical Model of Mind-Brain Interaction," *Philosophical Transactions of the Royal Society of London, Series B, Biological Sciences* 360, no. 1458 (2005): 1309–27; Jeffrey M. Schwartz and Sharon Begley, *The Mind and the Brain: Neuroplasticity and the Power of Mental Force* (New York: Harper, 2003), 27; William R. Uttal, "The Two Faces of MRI," *Cerebrum*, July 1, 2002, http://www.dana.org/Cerebrum/Default.aspx?id=39300; Wellcome Trust, "Brain's Architecture Makes Our View of the World Unique," *ScienceDaily*, December 6, 2010, www.sciencedaily.com/releases/2010/12/101205202512.htm; J. Richard Middleton, *The Liberating Image: The Imago Dei in Genesis 1* (Grand Rapids: Brazos, 2005); A. G. Christy et al., "Straying from the Righteous Path and from Ourselves: The Interplay between Perceptions of Morality and Self-Knowledge," *Personality and Social Psychology Bulletin* 1, no. 42 (2016): 1538–50; F. Gino et al., "The Moral Virtue of Authenticity," *Psychological Science* 26, no. 7 (2015): 983–86; Peter Kinderman, *The New Laws of Psychology: Why Nature and Nurture Alone Can't Explain Human Behavior* (London: Robinson, 2014).
34. Ibid.
35. Ibid.
36. Leaf, "The Mind Mapping Approach: A Model and Framework for Geodesic Learning."

Chapter 18 The Gift Profile

1. Stuart Hameroff and Roger Penrose, "Consciousness in the Universe: A Review of the 'Orch OR' Theory," *Physics of Life Reviews* 11, no. 1 (2014): 39–78; Stuart Hameroff et al., "Conduction Pathways in Microtubules, Biological Quantum Computation, and Consciousness," *Biosystems* 64, no. 1 (2002): 149–68; Stuart Hameroff, "Consciousness, Microtubules, and 'Orch OR': A 'Space-Time Odyssey,'" *Journal of*

Consciousness Studies 21, nos. 3–4 (2014): 126–53; Stuart Hameroff, "How Quantum Brain Biology Can Rescue Conscious Free Will," *Frontiers in Integrative Neuroscience* 6 (2012); Stuart R. Hameroff, Alfred W. Kaszniak, and Alwyn Scott, eds. *Toward a Science of Consciousness II: The Second Tucson Discussions and Debates*, vol. 2 (Cambridge, MA: MIT Press, 1998); Stuart R. Hameroff and Roger Penrose, "Conscious Events as Orchestrated Space-Time Selections," *Journal of Consciousness Studies* 3, no. 1 (1996): 36–53; Roger Penrose, *Shadows of the Mind*, vol. 4 (Oxford: Oxford University Press, 1994); Scott Hagan, Stuart R. Hameroff, and Jack A. Tuszyński, "Quantum Computation in Brain Microtubules: Decoherence and Biological Feasibility," *Physical Review E* 65, no. 6 (2002), doi:10.1103/PhysRevE.65.061901; Stuart Hameroff and Roger Penrose, "Consciousness in the Universe: An Updated Review of the 'Orch OR' Theory," *Biophysics of Consciousness: A Foundational Approach*, edited by R. R. Poznanski, J. A. Tuszynski, and T. E. Feinberg (Singapore: World Scientific, 2016); Satyajit Sahu et al., "Computational Myths and Mysteries That Have Grown around Microtubule in the Last Half a Century and Their Possible Verification," *Journal of Computational and Theoretical Nanoscience* 8, no. 3 (2011): 509–15.

2. Ibid.

3. Hameroff and Penrose, "Consciousness in the Universe: An Updated Review of the 'Orch OR' Theory;" Satyajit Sahu et al., "Computational Myths and Mysteries."

4. Estimates of the number of thoughts we think in a day vary widely. For example, Charlie Greer writes, "Several years ago, the National Science Foundation put out some very interesting statistics. We think a thousand thoughts per hour. When we write, we think twenty-five hundred thoughts in an hour and a half. The average person thinks about twelve thousand thoughts per day. A deeper thinker, according to this report, puts forth fifty thousand thoughts daily." See Charlie Greer, "What Are You Thinking, Part Deux," Charlie Greer's HVAC Profit Boosters, Inc., accessed January 25, 2018, http://www.hvacprofitboosters.com/Tips/Tip_Archive/tip_archive7.html.

5. Leaf, "The Mind Mapping Approach: A Model and Framework for Geodesic Learning;" Leaf, "The Development of a Model for Geodesic Learning: The Geodesic Information Processing Model;" C. M. Leaf, I. C. Uys, and B. Louw, "An Alternative Non-Traditional Approach to Learning: The Metacognitive-Mapping Approach;" Asael Y. Sklar et al., "Reading and Doing Arithmetic Nonconsciously," *Proceedings of the National Academy of Sciences* 109, no. 48 (2012): 19614–19.

6. Ibid.

7. Harold Pashler et al., "Learning Styles: Concepts and Evidence," *Psychological Science in the Public Interest* 9, no. 3 (2008): 105–19.; Lynn Curry, "A Critique of the Research on Learning Styles," *Educational Leadership* 48, no. 2 (1990): 50–56; Frank Coffield et al., *Learning Styles and Pedagogy in Post-16 Learning: A Systematic and Critical Review*, (London: Learning Skills and Research Centre, 2004), http://www.leerbeleving.nl/wp-content/uploads/2011/09/learning-styles.pdf; Paul A. Kirschner, "Stop Propagating the Learning Styles Myth," *Computers & Education* 106 (2017): 166–71.

8. Ibid.

9. Pashler et al., "Learning Styles: Concepts and Evidence;" Leaf, "The Development of a Model for Geodesic Learning: The Geodesic Information Processing Model;" Leaf, "An Altered Perception of Learning: Geodesic Learning: Part 2," *Therapy Africa* 2, no. 1 (January/February 1998): 4; Curry, "A Critique of the Research on Learning Styles;" Doug Rohrer and Harold Pashler, "Learning Styles: Where's the Evidence?"

Online Submission 46, no. 7 (2012): 634–35; Kirschner, "Stop Propagating the Learning Styles Myth."

10. Philip M. Newton, "The Learning Styles Myth Is Thriving in Higher Education," *Frontiers in Psychology* 6 (2015): 1908; Philip M. Newton and Mahallad Miah, "Evidence-Based Higher Education: Is the Learning Styles 'Myth' Important?" *Frontiers in Psychology* 8 (2017): 444.

11. Ron Finley, "A Guerilla Gardener in South Central LA," YouTube video, uploaded by TED on March 6, 2013, https://www.youtube.com/watch?v=EzZzZ_qpZ4w.

12. For the more comprehensive profile, see the Perfectly You app, www.perfectly you.com.

Chapter 19 Characteristics of the Seven Modules

1. Binghamton University, "Researchers Can Identify You by Your Brain Waves with 100 Percent Accuracy;" Maria V. Ruiz-Blondet et al., "A Novel Method for Very High Accuracy Event-Related Potential Biometric Identification."

2. Weizmann Institute of Science, "Smell Fingerprints?"

3. D. Samuel Schwarzkopf, Chen Song, and Geraint Rees, "The Surface Area of Human V1 Predicts the Subjective Experience of Object Size," *Nature Neuroscience* 14, no. 1 (2011): 28–30; Wellcome Trust, "Brain's Architecture Makes Our View of the World Unique," *ScienceDaily*, Dec. 6, 2010, www.sciencedaily.com/releases/2010/12/101205202512.htm.; Ryota Kanai and Geraint Rees, "The Structural Basis of Inter-Individual Differences in Human Behaviour and Cognition," *Nature Reviews Neuroscience* 12, no. 4 (2011): 231–42; Aaron Alexander-Bloch, Jay N. Giedd, and Ed Bullmore, "Imaging Structural Co-variance between Human Brain Regions," *Nature Reviews Neuroscience* 14, no. 5 (2013): 322–36; Mariko Osaka et al., "The Neural Basis of Individual Differences in Working Memory Capacity: An fMRI Study," *NeuroImage* 18, no. 3 (2003): 789–97; Edward K. Vogel and Edward Awh, "How to Exploit Diversity for Scientific Gain: Using Individual Differences to Constrain Cognitive Theory," *Current Directions in Psychological Science* 17, no. 2 (2008): 171–76.

4. Moran Gershoni and Shmuel Pietrokovski, "The Landscape of Sex-Differential Transcriptome and Its Consequent Selection in Human Adults," *BMC Biology* 15, no. 1 (2017): 7; J. Cairns et al., "The Origin of Mutants," *Nature* 35 (1988): 142–45.

Chapter 20 What Is Learning?

1. Willoughby B. Britton et al., "Dismantling Mindfulness-Based Cognitive Therapy: Creation and Validation of 8-Week Focused Attention and Open Monitoring Interventions within a 3-Armed Randomized Controlled Trial," *Behaviour Research and Therapy* (2017), doi:10.1016/j.brat.2017.09.010; Georgetown University Medical Center, "Mindfulness Meditation Training Lowers Biomarkers of Stress Response in Anxiety Disorder: Hormonal, Inflammatory Reactions to Stress Were Reduced after Meditation Training, in Rigorous NIH-Sponsored Trial," press release, January 24, 2017, https://gumc.georgetown.edu/news/mindfulness-meditation-training-lowers-biomarkers-of-stress-response-in-anxiety-disorder; Yi-Yuan Tang, Britta K. Hölzel, and Michael I. Posner, "The Neuroscience of Mindfulness Meditation," *Nature Reviews Neuroscience* 16, no. 4 (2015): 213–25.

2. Benjamin C. Storm, Sean M. Stone, and Aaron S. Benjamin, "Using the Internet to Access Information Inflates Future Use of the Internet to Access Other Information," *Memory* 25, no. 6 (2017): 717–23; Amanda M. Ferguson, David McLean, and Evan F. Risko, "Answers at Your Fingertips: Access to the Internet Influences Willingness to Answer Questions," *Consciousness and Cognition* 37 (2015): 91–102; James W. Antony et al., "Retrieval as a Fast Route to Memory Consolidation," *Trends in Cognitive Sciences* 21, no. 8 (2017): 573–76; Ekaterina Haskins, "Between Archive and Participation: Public Memory in a Digital Age," *Rhetoric Society Quarterly* 37, no. 4 (2007): 401–22; Maria Wimber et al., "Prefrontal Dopamine and the Dynamic Control of Human Long-Term Memory," *Translational Psychiatry* 1, no. 7 (2011): e15; Kaspersky Lab, "The Rise and Impact of Digital Amnesia: Why We Need to Protect What We No Longer Remember," accessed January 25, 2018, https://d1srlirzdlmpew .cloudfront.net/wp-content/uploads/sites/92/2017/06/06024645/005-Kaspersky-Digital -Amnesia-19.6.15.pdf.

3. Evan F. Risko and Sam J. Gilbert, "Cognitive Offloading," *Trends in Cognitive Sciences* 20, no. 9 (2016): 676–88; Storm, Stone, and Benjamin, "Using the Internet to Access Information;" Ferguson, McLean, and Risko, "Answers at Your Fingertips."

4. Stuart Wolpert, "Is Technology Producing a Decline in Critical Thinking and Analysis?" *UCLA Newsroom*, January 27, 2009, http://newsroom.ucla.edu/releases/ is-technology-producing-a-decline-79127; Steven Gerardi, "Use of Computers/Apps and the Negative Effects on Children's Intellectual Outcomes," *Sociology* 7 (2017): 128–32; Zhanna Bagdasarov, Yupeng Luo, and Wei Wu, "The Influence of Tablet-Based Technology on the Development of Communication and Critical Thinking Skills: An Interdisciplinary Study," *Journal of Research on Technology in Education* 49, no. 1–2 (2017): 55–72.

5. James Schroeder, "More Bad News about Smartphones: When Will We Heed the Warnings?" *Mad in America*, November 12, 2017, https://www.madinamerica .com/2017/11/bad-news-about-smartphones/.

6. Ibid.

7. Rob Price, "Billionaire Ex-Facebook President Sean Parker Unloads on Mark Zuckerberg and Admits He Helped Build a Monster," *Business Insider*, November 9, 2017, http://www.businessinsider.com/ex-facebook-president-sean-parker-social-ne twork-human-vulnerability-2017-11.

8. Travis J. A. Craddock, Jack A. Tuszynski, and Stuart Hameroff, "Cytoskeletal Signaling: Is Memory Encoded in Microtubule Lattices by CaMKII Phosphorylation?" *PLoS Computational Biology* 8, no. 3 (2012): e1002421; Hameroff and Penrose, "Consciousness in the Universe: A Review of the 'Orch OR' Theory"; Emmanuel M. Pothos and Jerome R. Busemeyer, "Can Quantum Probability Provide a New Direction for Cognitive Modeling?" *Behavioral and Brain Sciences* 36, no. 3 (2013): 255–74; Hameroff, "How Quantum Brain Biology Can Rescue Conscious Free Will;" Diederik Aerts et al., "Quantum Structure and Human Thought," *Behavioral and Brain Sciences* 36, no. 3 (2013): 274–76; Gary L. Brase and James Shanteau, "The Unbearable Lightness of 'Thinking': Moving beyond Simple Concepts of Thinking, Rationality, and Hypothesis Testing," *Behavioral and Brain Sciences* 34, no. 5 (2011): 250–51.

9. George Kastellakis et al., "Synaptic Clustering within Dendrites: An Emerging Theory of Memory Formation," *Progress in Neurobiology* 126 (2015): 19–35.

10. Leaf, "Mind Mapping."

11. Leaf, "The Mind Mapping Approach."

12. Carol Dweck, "Implicit Theories of Intelligence Predict Achievement across Adolescent Transition: A Longitudinal Study and an Intervention," *Child Development* 78 (2007): 246–63.

13. Alvaro Pascual-Leone et al., "Modulation of Muscle Responses Evoked by Transcranial Magnetic Stimulation during the Acquisition of New Fine Motor Skills," *Journal of Neurophysiology* 74, no. 3 (1995): 1037–45; Sharon Begley, "The Brain: How the Brain Rewires Itself," *Time*, January 19, 2007, http://content.time.com/time /magazine/article/0,9171,1580438,00.html.

14. Mégane Missaire et al., "Long-Term Effects of Interference on Short-Term Memory Performance in the Rat," *PloS one* 12, no. 3 (2017): e0173834; Jan Kamiński, Aneta Brzezicka, and Andrzej Wróbel, "Short-Term Memory Capacity (7±2) Predicted by Theta to Gamma Cycle Length Ratio," *Neurobiology of Learning and Memory* 95, no. 1 (2011): 19–23; John E. Lisman and Ole Jensen, "The Theta-Gamma Neural Code," *Neuron* 77, no. 6 (2013): 1002–16; James Clear, "How Long Does It Actually Take to Form a New Habit? (Backed by Science)," *James Clear*, accessed January 25, 2018, https://jamesclear.com/new-habit.

Chapter 21 What Is Memory?

1. "The Nobel Prize in Physiology or Medicine 1906," Nobelprize.org, accessed January 25, 2018, https://www.nobelprize.org/nobel_prizes/medicine/laureates/1906/.

2. Raymond M. Klein, "The Hebb Legacy," *Canadian Journal of Experimental Psychology/Revue canadienne de psychologie expérimentale* 53, no. 1 (1999): 1; Bonnie Strickland, ed., "Hebb, Donald O. (1904–1985)," *Gale Encyclopedia of Psychology*, second ed. (Farmington Hills, MI: Gale Group, 2001).

3. Mark E. J. Sheffield and Daniel A. Dombeck, "Calcium Transient Prevalence across the Dendritic Arbour Predicts Place Field Properties," *Nature* 517, no. 7533 (2015): 200–204; Trygve Solstad, Edvard I. Moser, and Gaute T. Einevoll, "From Grid Cells to Place Cells: A Mathematical Model," *Hippocampus* 16, no. 12 (2006): 1026–31.

4. Craddock, Tuszynski, and Hameroff, "Cytoskeletal Signaling;" John Lisman, "The CaM Kinase II Hypothesis for the Storage of Synaptic Memory," *Trends in Neurosciences* 17, no. 10 (1994): 406–12; Hameroff et al., "Conduction Pathways in Microtubules;" Leif Dehmelt and Shelley Halpain, "The MAP2/Tau Family of Microtubule-Associated Proteins," *Genome Biology* 6, no. 1 (2004): 204; Akihiro Harada et al., "MAP2 Is Required for Dendrite Elongation, PKA Anchoring in Dendrites, and Proper PKA Signal Transduction," *J Cell Biol* 158, no. 3 (2002): 541–49; Jacek Jaworski et al., "Dynamic Microtubules Regulate Dendritic Spine Morphology and Synaptic Plasticity," *Neuron* 61, no. 1 (2009): 85–100; Nicolas Toni et al., "LTP Promotes Formation of Multiple Spine Synapses between a Single Axon Terminal and a Dendrite," *Nature* 402, no. 6760 (1999): 421–25; Stuart R. Hameroff and Richard C. Watt, "Information Processing in Microtubules," *Journal of Theoretical Biology* 98, no. 4 (1982): 549–61; N. J. Woolf, A. Priel, and J. A. Tuszynski, *Nanoneuroscience* (Berlin: Springer, 2010); N. J. Woolf, "Microtubules in the Cerebral Cortex: Role in Memory and Consciousness," J. A. Tuszynski, ed., *The Emerging Physics of Consciousness* (Berlin: Springer, 2006), 49–94; C. Sanchez, J. Diaz-Nido, and J. Avila, "Phosphorylation of Microtubule-Associated Protein 2 (MAP2) and Its Relevance for the Regulation of the

Neuronal Cytoskeleton Function," *Progress in Neurobiology* 61, no. 2 (2000): 133–68; John Cronly-Dillon, David Carden, and Carole Berks, "The Possible Involvement of Brain Microtubules in Memory Fixation," *Journal of Experimental Biology* 61, no. 2 (1974): 443–54; Nancy J. Woolf, Marcus D. Zinnerman, and Gail V. W. Johnson, "Hippocampal Microtubule-Associated Protein-2 Alterations with Contextual Memory," *Brain Research* 821, no. 1 (1999): 241–49; Stuart Hameroff, "The 'Conscious Pilot'— Dendritic Synchrony Moves through the Brain to Mediate Consciousness," *Journal of Biological Physics* 36, no. 1 (2010): 71–93.

5. Panayiota Poirazi and Bartlett W. Mel, "Impact of Active Dendrites and Structural Plasticity on the Memory Capacity of Neural Tissue," *Neuron* 29, no. 3 (2001): 779–96; Attila Losonczy, Judit K. Makara, and Jeffrey C. Magee, "Compartmentalized Dendritic Plasticity and Input Feature Storage in Neurons," *Nature* 452, no. 7186 (2008): 436–41; Matthew E. Larkum and Thomas Nevian, "Synaptic Clustering by Dendritic Signalling Mechanisms," *Current Opinion in Neurobiology* 18, no. 3 (2008): 321–31; Kevin A. Archie and Bartlett W. Mel, "A Model for Intradendritic Computation of Binocular Disparity," *Nature Neuroscience* 3, no. 1 (2000): 54–63; Dmitri B. Chklovskii, B. W. Mel, and K. Svoboda, "Cortical Rewiring and Information Storage," *Nature* 431, no. 7010 (2004): 782–88; P. Jesper Sjöström et al., "Dendritic Excitability and Synaptic Plasticity," *Physiological Reviews* 88, no. 2 (2008): 769–840; Bartlett W. Mel, Jackie Schiller, and Panayiota Poirazi, "Synaptic Plasticity in Dendrites: Complications and Coping Strategies," *Current Opinion in Neurobiology* 43 (2017): 177–86; Ju Lu and Yi Zuo, "Clustered Structural and Functional Plasticity of Dendritic Spines," *Brain Research Bulletin* 129 (2017): 18–22; Jacopo Bono and Claudia Clopath, "Modeling Somatic and Dendritic Spike Mediated Plasticity at the Single Neuron and Network Level," *Nature Communications* 8, no. 1 (2017): 706; Tobias Bonhoeffer and Pico Caroni, "Structural Plasticity in Dendrites and Spines," *Dendrites*, edited by Greg Stuart, Nelson Spruston, and Michael Häusser (Oxford: Oxford University Press, 2016), 557–79.

6. Craddock, Tuszynski, and Hameroff, "Cytoskeletal Signaling;" Stuart Hameroff, "How Quantum Brain Biology Can Rescue Conscious Free Will;" Jerome R. Busemeyer, J. Wang, and Richard M. Shiffrin, "Bayesian Model Comparison of Quantum Versus Traditional Models of Decision Making for Explaining Violations of the Dynamic Consistency Principle," paper presented at Foundations and Applications of Utility, Risk and Decision Theory Conference, June 2012, Atlanta, Georgia; Brase and Shanteau, "The Unbearable Lightness of 'Thinking';" Hameroff and Penrose, "Consciousness in the Universe: A Review of the 'Orch OR' Theory"; Emmanuel M. Pothos and Jerome R. Busemeyer, "Can Quantum Probability Provide a New Direction for Cognitive Modeling?" *Behavioral and Brain Sciences* 36, no. 3 (2013): 255–74; Diederik Aerts et al., "Quantum Structure and Human Thought," *Behavioral and Brain Sciences* 36, no. 3 (2013): 274–76; Bridget N. Queenan et al., "On the Research of Time Past: The Hunt for the Substrate of Memory," *Annals of the New York Academy of Sciences* 1396, no. 1 (2017): 108–25.

7. Ibid.

8. Henry P. Stapp, *Mindful Universe: Quantum Mechanics and the Participating Observer* (Berlin: Springer, 2011), Kindle loc. 316; Stapp, *Mind, Matter and Quantum Mechanics*, Kindle loc. 687, 694, 1783–84.

9. Poirazi and Mel, "Impact of Active Dendrites and Structural Plasticity;" Losonczy, Makara, and Magee, "Compartmentalized Dendritic Plasticity and Input Feature

Storage in Neurons;" Jackie Schiller et al., "NMDA Spikes in Basal Dendrites of Cortical Pyramidal Neurons," *Nature* 404, no. 6775 (2000): 285–89; Jacopo Bono, Katharina A. Wilmes, and Claudia Clopath, "Modelling Plasticity in Dendrites: From Single Cells to Networks," *Current Opinion in Neurobiology* 46 (2017): 136–41; Mel, Schiller, and Poirazi, "Synaptic Plasticity in Dendrites."

10. Michael Häusser, "Storing Memories in Dendritic Channels," *Nature Neuroscience* 7, no. 2 (2004): 98–100; Andreas Frick and Daniel Johnston, "Plasticity of Dendritic Excitability," *Developmental Neurobiology* 64, no. 1 (2005): 100–115; Bono, Wilmes, and Clopath, "Modelling Plasticity in Dendrites."

11. Stapp, *Mind, Matter and Quantum Mechanics*, Kindle loc. 2958, 2972–76.

12. P. C. W. Davies and Neils Hendrik Gregersen, *Information and the Nature of Reality: From Physics to Metaphysics* (Cambridge, UK: Cambridge University Press, 2010), 85.

13. Stapp, *Mind, Matter and Quantum Mechanics*, Kindle loc. 1729.

14. Häusser, "Storing Memories in Dendritic Channels;" Frick and Johnston, "Plasticity of Dendritic Excitability;" Bono, Wilmes, and Clopath, "Modelling Plasticity in Dendrites."

15. Travis J. A. Craddock, Stuart R. Hameroff, and Jack A. Tuszynski, "The Quantum Underground: Where Life and Consciousness Originate," *Biophysics of Consciousness: A Foundational Approach*, edited by Roman R. Poznanski, Jack Tusnynski, and Todd E. Feinberg (Singapore: World Scientific, 2016), 459–515.

16. Craddock, Tuszynski, and Hameroff, "Cytoskeletal Signaling."

17. Stapp, *Mind, Matter and Quantum Mechanics*, Kindle loc. 64, 75–77; Harald Atmanspacher, "Quantum Approaches to Brain and Mind," *The Blackwell Companion to Consciousness*, edited by Max Velmans and Susan Schneider (Hoboken, NJ: Blackwell Publishing, 2017), 298; Henry P. Stapp, "Mind, Matter, and Quantum Mechanics," *Foundations of Physics* 12, no. 4 (1982): 363–99; Stuart Hameroff, "Consciousness, Neurobiology and Quantum Mechanics: The Case for a Connection," *The Emerging Physics of Consciousness*, edited by Jack A. Tuszynski (Berlin: Springer, 2006), 193–253; Penrose, *The Emperor's New Mind*; Amit Goswami, "Consciousness in Quantum Physics and the Mind-Body Problem," *The Journal of Mind and Behavior* (1990): 75–96; Stapp, "A Quantum Theory of Consciousness," *Mind, Matter and Quantum Mechanics*, 39–47; Stuart Hameroff and Roger Penrose, "Orchestrated Reduction of Quantum Coherence in Brain Microtubules: A Model for Consciousness," *Mathematics and Computers in Simulation* 40, no. 3–4 (1996): 453–80.

18. Stapp, *Mind, Matter and Quantum Mechanics*, Kindle loc. 2976, 2980.

19. Hameroff, "Consciousness, Neurobiology and Quantum Mechanics."

20. Stapp, *Mind, Matter and Quantum Mechanics*, Kindle loc. 2193, 2200.

21. Erich Joos et al., *Decoherence and the Appearance of a Classical World in Quantum Theory* (Berlin: Springer, 2013); Stapp, *Mind, Matter and Quantum Mechanics*, Kindle loc. 3092, 3297.

22. Christopher A. Fuchs, "Distinguishability and Accessible Information in Quantum Theory," Cornell University Library, January 23, 1996, https://arxiv.org/abs/quant-ph/9601020.

23. Stapp, *Mind, Matter and Quantum Mechanics*, Kindle loc. 40, 1729, 3014; Henry Stapp, "Quantum Interactive Dualism: An Alternative to Materialism," *Journal*

of Consciousness Studies 12, no. 11 (2005): 43–58; Lucio Tonello and Massimo Cocchi, "The Cell Membrane: Is It a Bridge from Psychiatry to Quantum Consciousness?" *NeuroQuantology* 8, no. 1 (2010) 54–60.

24. Mark R. Rosenzweig, Edward L. Bennett, and Marian Cleeves Diamond, "Brain Changes in Response to Experience," *Scientific American* 226, no. 2 (1972): 22–29; A. M. Clare Kelly and Hugh Garavan, "Human Functional Neuroimaging of Brain Changes Associated with Practice," *Cerebral Cortex* 15, no. 8 (2004): 1089–102; David Krech, Mark R. Rosenzweig, and Edward L. Bennett, "Relations between Brain Chemistry and Problem-Solving among Rats Raised in Enriched and Impoverished Environments," *Journal of Comparative and Physiological Psychology* 55, no. 5 (1962): 801; M. C. Diamond, "The Significance of Enrichment," *Enriching Heredity* (New York: Free Press, 1988); Marian Cleeves Diamond, "What Are the Determinants of Children's Academic Successes and Difficulties?" *New Horizons for Learning*, accessed January 25, 2018, http://archive.education.jhu.edu/PD/newhorizons/Neurosciences/articles/Determinants%20of%20Academic%20Success%20and%20Difficulties/index.ht ml; M. C. Diamond, "The Brain . . . Use It or Lose It," *Mindshift Connection* 1, no. 1 (1996): 1; Marian Diamond and Janet Hopson, *Magic Trees of the Mind: How to Nurture your Child's Intelligence, Creativity, and Healthy Emotions from Birth Through Adolescence* (New York: Penguin, 1999).

25. Qiang Zhou, Koichi J. Homma, and Mu-ming Poo, "Shrinkage of Dendritic Spines Associated with Long-Term Depression of Hippocampal Synapses," *Neuron* 44, no. 5 (2004): 749–57; Masao Ito, "Long-Term Depression," *Annual Review of Neuroscience* 12, no. 1 (1989): 85–102.

26. Mégane Missaire et al., "Long-Term Effects of Interference on Short-Term Memory Performance in the Rat;" Kamiński, Brzezicka, and Wróbel, "Short-Term Memory Capacity (7±2) Predicted by Theta to Gamma Cycle Length Ratio;" John E. Lisman and Ole Jensen, "The Theta-Gamma Neural Code," *Neuron* 77, no. 6 (2013): 1002–16; Clear, "How Long Does It Actually Take to Form a New Habit?"

27. Lally et al., "How Are Habits Formed;" Sheina Orbell and Bas Verplanken, "The Automatic Component of Habit in Health Behavior: Habit as Cue-Contingent Automaticity," *Health Psychology* 29, no. 4 (2010): 374; Phillippa Lally and Benjamin Gardner, "Promoting Habit Formation," *Health Psychology Review* 7, no. sup1 (2013): S137–S158; Lally, Wardle, and Gardner, "Experiences of Habit Formation;" Wendy Wood and David T. Neal, "A New Look at Habits and the Habit-Goal Interface," *Psychological Review* 114, no. 4 (2007): 843; Wendy Wood, Leona Tam, and Melissa Guerrero Witt, "Changing Circumstances, Disrupting Habits," *Journal of Personality and Social Psychology* 88, no. 6 (2005): 918; David T. Neal et al., "The Pull of the Past: When Do Habits Persist despite Conflict with Motives?" *Personality and Social Psychology Bulletin* 37, no. 11 (2011): 1428–37; Benjamin Gardner, "A Review and Analysis of the Use of 'Habit' in Understanding, Predicting and Influencing Health-Related Behaviour," *Health Psychology Review* 9, no. 3 (2015): 277–95; Marion Fournier et al., "Effects of Circadian Cortisol on the Development of a Health Habit," *Health Psychology* 36, no. 11 (2017): 1059; Justin O'Hare, Nicole Calakos, and Henry H. Yin, "Recent Insights into Corticostriatal Circuit Mechanisms Underlying Habits," *Current Opinion in Behavioral Sciences* 20 (2018): 40–46; Sheffield and Dombeck, "Calcium Transient Prevalence across the Dendritic Arbour."

28. See my other books and programs for more information on this process, such as *Switch On Your Brain*, *Think and Eat Yourself Smart*, and *The Perfect You*.

29. Maya Frankfurt and Victoria Luine, "The Evolving Role of Dendritic Spines and Memory: Interaction(s) with Estradiol," *Hormones and Behavior* 74 (2015): 28–36; Diamond, "The Significance of Enrichment;" Diamond, "The Brain . . . Use It or Lose It;" Diamond and Hopson, *Magic Trees of the Mind*; Karyn M. Frick et al., "Sex Steroid Hormones Matter for Learning and Memory: Estrogenic Regulation of Hippocampal Function in Male and Female Rodents," *Learning & Memory* 22, no. 9 (2015): 472–93; C. D. Gipson and M. F. Olive, "Structural and Functional Plasticity of Dendritic Spines—Root or Result of Behavior?" *Genes, Brain and Behavior* 16, no. 1 (2017): 101–17; Maria-Angeles Arevalo et al., "Signaling Mechanisms Mediating the Regulation of Synaptic Plasticity and Memory by Estradiol," *Hormones and Behavior* 74 (2015): 19–27.

30. Craddock, Tuszynski, and Hameroff, "Cytoskeletal Signaling;" Hameroff and Penrose, "Consciousness in the Universe: A Review of the 'Orch OR' Theory;" Emmanuel M. Pothos and Jerome R. Busemeyer, "Can Quantum Probability Provide a New Direction for Cognitive Modeling?" *Behavioral and Brain Sciences* 36, no. 3 (2013): 255–74; Hameroff, "How Quantum Brain Biology Can Rescue Conscious Free Will;" Diederik Aerts et al., "Quantum Structure and Human Thought," *Behavioral and Brain Sciences* 36, no. 3 (2013): 274–76; Brase and Shanteau, "The Unbearable Lightness of 'Thinking'."

31. Ibid.

32. Ibid.

33. Ibid.

34. Ibid.

35. Ibid.

36. Ibid.

37. Ibid.

38. Ibid.

39. Ibid.

40. Ibid.

41. Jeffrey Mishlove, "Consciousness and the Brain, Part Four: The Orchestra of the Brain, with Stuart Hameroff," YouTube video, uploaded by New Thinking Allowed, August 18, 2015, https://m.youtube.com/watch?v=hHDfGAnDedw; Jeffrey Mishlove, "Consciousness and the Brain, Part Five: Consciousness in the Universe, with Stuart Hameroff," New Thinking Allowed, YouTube video, August 19, 2015, https://m.youtube.com/watch?v=W9V3Ht1jnCU; Jeffrey Mishlove, "Consciousness and the Brain, Part Six: Spiritual Implications, with Stuart Hameroff," YouTube video, uploaded by New Thinking Allowed, August 20, 2015, https://m.youtube.com/watch?v=jPlBGdZLwTE.

42. Henry Stapp, "Minds and Values in the Quantum Universe," *Information and the Nature of Reality from Physics to Metaphysics*, edited by P. C. W. Davies and Niels Henrik Gregersen (Cambridge, UK: Cambridge University Press, 2014): 157.

43. Stapp, "Quantum Interactive-Dualism."

44. Werner Heisenberg, *Physics and Philosophy: The Revolution in Modern Science* (New York: Harper and Row, 1958); David C. Cassidy, *Werner Heisenberg: A Bibliography of His Writings*, second ed. (New York: Whittier, 2001).

45. John von Neumann, *Mathematical Foundations of Quantum Mechanics*, trans. Robert T. Beyer (Princeton: Princeton University Press, 1955).

46. Ibid.

47. Stapp, "Quantum Interactive-Dualism."

48. Schwartz, Stapp, and Beauregard, "Quantum Physics in Neuroscience and Psychology."

49. Keith Ward, "Keith Ward—The New Atheists, Part 1," YouTube video, uploaded by ObjectiveBob, August 29, 2012, https://www.youtube.com/watch?v=fkJshx-7l5w.

50. J. S. Bell, *Speakable and Unspeakable in Quantum Mechanics: Collected Papers on Quantum Philosophy* (Cambridge, UK: Cambridge University Press, 2004).

Chapter 22 The Geodesic Information Processing Theory

1. Bell, *Speakable and Unspeakable*.

2. H. Gardner, *Frames of Mind* (New York: Basic Books, 2011); J. M. Shine et al., "The Dynamics of Functional Brain Networks: Integrated Network States during Cognitive Task Performance," *Neuron* 92, no. 2 (October 19, 2016): 544–54.

3. Leaf, *Switch On Your Brain*; Lally et al., "How Are Habits Formed;" Clear, "How Long Does It Actually Take to Form a New Habit?"

4. B. Libet, "Do We Have Free Will?" *Journal of Consciousness Studies*, 6, nos. 8–9 (1999): 47–57.

5. C. S. Soon, "Unconscious Determinants of Free Decisions in the Human Brain," *Nature Neuroscience* 11, no. 5 (April 13, 2008): 543–45.

6. "Libet Experiments," *The Information Philosopher*, accessed January 18, 2018, http://www.informationphilosopher.com/freedom/libet_experiments.html.

7. C. S. Herrmann et al., "Analysis of a Choice-Reaction Task Yields a New Interpretation of Libet's Experiments," *International Journal of Psychophysiology* 67 (2008): 156, http://www.fflch.usp.br/df/opessoa/Hermann%20-%20New%20interpretation%20-%20%202008.pdf.

8. Ibid.

9. Benjamin Libet, *Mind Time: The Temporal Factor in Consciousness* (Cambridge, MA: Harvard University Press, 2004).

10. D. Denett et al., *Neuroscience and Philosophy: Brain, Mind, and Language* (New York: Columbia University Press, 2007).

11. Shira Sardi et al., "Adaptive Nodes Enrich Nonlinear Cooperative Learning beyond Traditional Adaptation by Links," *Scientific Reports* 8 (2018): 1–10.

Recommended Reading

The concepts I teach in this book cover a wide spectrum and include years of reading, researching, and working with clients in my private practice, in schools, in churches, and in corporations. If I had to provide all the citations I have used over the past thirty years, there would be almost as many citations as words! Since this book is intended for a popular audience, I have included the principal sources that have shaped my thinking in order to communicate my message as effectively as I can.

The book list that follows is less of a bibliography (which would also be too long) and more of a recommended reading list of some of my favorite books, scientific articles, and other resources I have used over the years, and still use. I hope you love them as much as I do!

Adams, H. B., and B. Wallace. "A Model for Curriculum Development: TASC." *Gifted Education International* 7 (1991): 194–213.

Alavi, A., and L. J. Hirsch. "Studies of Central Nervous System Disorders with Single Photon Emission Computed Tomography and Positron Emission Tomography: Evolution Over the Past 2 Decades." *Seminars in Nuclear Medicine* 21, no. 1 (January 1991): 51–58.

Alesandrini, K. L. "Imagery: Eliciting Strategies and Meaningful Learning." *Journal of Educational Psychology* 62 (1982): 526–30.

Allport, D. A. "Patterns and Actions: Cognitive Mechanisms and Content Specific." In *Cognitive Psychology: New Directions*, edited by G. L. Claxton. London: Routledge & Kegan Paul, 1980.

Amen, D. G. *Change Your Brain, Change Your Life*. New York: Three Rivers Press, 1998.

———. *Magnificent Mind at Any Age*. New York: Harmony Books, 2008.

Amend, A. E. "Defining and Demystifying Baroque, Classic and Romantic Music." *Journal of the Society for Accelerative Learning and Teaching* 14, no. 2 (1989): 91–112.

Amua-Quarshie, P. "Basalo-Cortical Interactions: The Role of the Basal Forebrain in Attention and Alzheimer's Disease." Unpublished Master's thesis. Newark: Rutgers University, 2009.

Anastasi, M. W., and A. B. Newberg. "A Preliminary Study of the Acute Effects of Religious Ritual on Anxiety." *The Journal of Alternative and Complementary Medicine* 14, no. 2 (March 2008): 163–65. doi:10.1089/acm.2007.0675.

Anderson, J. R. *Cognitive Psychology and Its Complications*. 2nd ed. New York: W. H. Freeman, 1985.

Arnheim, R. "Visual Thinking in Education." In *The Potential of Fantasy and Imagination*, edited by A. Sheikll and J. Shaffer, 215–25. New York: Brandon House, 1979.

Atkins, R. C. *Dr. Atkins Health Revolution*. Boston: Houghton Mifflin Company, 1990.

———. *Dr. Atkins New Diet Revolution*. London: Ebury Press, 2003.

———. *New Diet Cook Book*. London: Ebury Press, 2003.

Bach-y-Rita, P., et al. "Vision Substitution by Tactile Image Projection." *Nature* 221, no. 5184 (1969): 963–64.

Bancroft, W. J. "Accelerated Learning Techniques for the Foreign Language Classroom." *Per Linguam* 1, no. 2 (1985): 20–24.

Barker, J. A. *Discovering the Future: The Business of Paradigms*. Minneapolis: ILI Press, 1986.

Bartlett, F. C. *Remembering: A Study in Experimental and Social Psychology*. Cambridge, UK: Cambridge, 1932.

Baxter, R., S. B. Cohen, and M. Ylvisaker. "Comprehensive Cognitive Assessment." In *Head Injury Rehabilitation: Children and Adolescents*, edited by M. Ylvisaker, 247–75. San Diego: College-Hill Press, 1985.

Beauregard, M., and D. O'Leary. *The Spiritual Brain*. New York: Harper Collins, 2007.

Bereiter, L. "Toward a Solution of the Learning Paradox." *Review of Educational Research* 55 (1985): 201–25.

Berninger, V., A. Chen, and R. Abbot. "A Test of the Multiple Connections Model of Reading Acquisition." *International Journal of Neuroscience* 42 (1988): 283–95.

Bishop, J. H. "Why the Apathy in American High Schools?" *Educational Researcher* 18, no. 1 (1989): 6–10.

Block, N., and G. Dworkin. *The I.Q. Controversy*. New York: Pantheon, 1976.

Bloom, B. S. "The 2 Sigma Problem: The Search for Methods of Group Instruction as Effective as One-to-One Tutoring." *Educational Researcher* 13, no. 6 (1984): 4–16.

Bloom, F. E., ed. *The Best of the Brain from Scientific American: Mind, Matter and Tomorrow's Brain*. New York: Dana Press, 2007.

Bloom, F. E., et al., eds. *The Dana Guide to Brain Health*. New York: Dana Press, 2003.

Bloom, L., and M. Lahey. *Language Development and Language Disorders*. Mississauga, ON, Canada: Wiley & Sons, 1978.

Boller, K., and C. Rovee-Collier. "Contextual Coding and Recording of Infants' Memories." *Journal of Experimental Child Psychology* 53, no. 1 (1992): 1–23.

Borkowski, J. G., W. Schneider, and M. Pressley. "The Challenges of Teaching Good Information Processing to the Learning Disabled Student." *International Journal of Disability, Development and Education* 3, no. 3 (1989): 169–85.

Botha, L. "SALT in Practice: A Report on Progress." *Journal of the Society for Accelerative Learning and Teaching* 10, no. 3 (1985): 197–99.

Botkin, J. W., M. Elmandjra, and M. Malitza. *No Limits to Learning: Bridging the Human Gap; A Report to the Club of Rome.* New York: Pergamon Press, 1979.

Boyle, P. "Having a Higher Purpose in Life Reduces Risk of Death Among Older Adults." *(e)Science News* (June 15, 2009). http://escience news.com/articles/2009/06/15/having.a.higher.purpose.life.reduces .risk.death.among.older.adults.

"Brain and Mind Symposium." Columbia University (2004). http://c250. columbia.edu/c250_events/symposia/brain_mind/brain_mind_vid _archive.html.

Bransford, J. D. *Human Cognition.* Belmont, CA: Wadsworth, 1979.

Braten, I. "Vygotsky as Precursor to Metacognitive Theory, II: Vygotsky as Metacognitivist." *Scandinavian Journal of Educational Research* 35, no. 4 (1991): 305–20.

Braun, A. "The New Neuropsychology of Sleep Commentary." *Neuro-Psychoanalysis* 1 (1999): 196–201.

Briggs, M. H. "Team Talk: Communication Skills for Early Intervention Teams." *Journal of Childhood Communication Disorders* 15, no. 1 (1993): 33–40.

Broadbent, D. E. *Perception and Communication.* London: Pergamon Press, 1958.

Brown, A. L. "Knowing When, Where and How to Remember: A Problem of Meta-Cognition." In *Advances in Instructional Psychology,* edited by R. Glaser. Hillsdale, NJ: Lawrence/Erlbaum, 1978.

Bunker, V. J., W. M. McBurnett, and D. L. Fenimore. "Integrating Language Intervention throughout the School Community." *Journal of Childhood Communication Disorders* 11, no. 1 (1987): 185–92.

Buzan, T. *Head First.* London: Thorsons, 2000.

———. *Use Both Sides of Your Brain.* New York: Plume, 1991.

Buzan, T., and T. Dixon. *The Evolving Brain.* Exeter, UK: Wheaten & Co., 1976.

Buzan, T., and R. Keene. *The Age Heresy.* London: Ebury Press, 1996.

Bynum, J. *Matters of the Heart.* Lake Mary, FL: Charisma House, 2002.

Byron, R. *Behavior in Organizations: Understanding and Managing the Human Side of Work.* 2nd ed. Boston: Allyn & Bacon, 1986.

Byron, R., and D. Byrne. *Social Psychology: Understanding Human Interaction.* 4th ed. Boston: Allyn & Bacon, 1984.

Calvin, W., and G. Ojemann. *Conversations with Neil's Brain.* Reading, MA: Addison-Wesley, 1994.

Campbell, B., L. Campbell, and D. Dickinson. "Teaching and Learning through Multiple Intelligences." Seattle: New Horizons for Learning, 1992.

Campione, J. C., A. L. Brown, and N. R. Bryant. "Individual Differences in Learning and Memory." In *Human Abilities: An Information Processing Approach,* edited by R. J. Sternberg, 103–26. New York: West Freeman, 1985.

Capra, F. "The Turning Point: A New Vision of Reality." *The Futurist* 16, no. 6 (1982): 19–24.

Caskey, O. "Accelerating Concept Formation." *Journal of the Society for Accelerative Learning and Teaching* 11, no. 3 (1986): 137–45.

Chi, M. "Interactive Roles of Knowledge and Strategies in the Development of Organized Sorting and Recall." In *Thinking and Learning Skills* 2. Edited by S. F. Chipman, J. W. Segal, and R. Glaser. Hillsdale, NJ: Lawrence Erlbaum, 1985.

Childre, D., and H. Martin. *The Heartmath Solution.* San Francisco: HarperCollins, 1999.

Clancey, W. "Why Today's Computers Don't Learn the Way People Do." Paper presented at the Annual Meeting of the American Educational Research Association. Boston, MA, 1990.

Clark, A. J. "Forgiveness: A Neurological Model." *Medical Hypotheses* 65 (2005): 649–54.

Colbert, D. *The Bible Cure for Memory Loss.* Lake Mary, FL: Siloam Press, 2001.

———. *Deadly Emotions: Understand the Mind-Body-Spirit Connection that Can Heal or Destroy You.* Nashville: Thomas Nelson, 2003.

Concise Oxford Dictionary. 9th ed. Oxford: Oxford University Press, 1995.

Cook, N. D. "Colossal Inhibition: The Key to the Brain Code." *Behavioral Science* 29 (1984): 98–110.

Costa, A. L. "Mediating the Metacognitive." *Educational Leadership* 42, no. 3 (1984): 57–62.

Cousins, N. "Anatomy of an Illness as Perceived by the Patient." *New England Journal of Medicine* 295 (1976): 1458–63.

———. *Anatomy of an Illness as Perceived by the Patient.* New York: Bantam, 1981.

Crick, F. *The Astonishing Hypothesis: The Scientific Search for the Soul.* New York: Charles Scribner & Sons, 1979.

Crick, F. H. C. "Thinking about the Brain." *Scientific American* 241, no. 3 (1981): 228–49.

Cromie, William J. "Aging Brains Lose Less Than Thought." *Harvard University Gazette* (October 3, 1996). https://news.harvard.edu/gazette /1996/10.03/AgingBrainsLose.html.

Damasio, A. R. *The Feeling of What Happens: Body and Motion in the Making of Consciousness.* New York: Harcourt Brace, 1999.

Damico, J. S. "Addressing Language Concerns in the Schools: The SLP as Consultant." *Journal of Childhood Communication Disorders* 11, no. 1 (1987): 17–40.

Dartigues, J. F. "Use It or Lose It." *Omni* (February 1994): 34.

De Andrade, L. M. "Intelligence's Secret: The Limbic System and How to Mobilize It Through Suggestopedy." *Journal of the Society for Accelerative Learning and Teaching* 11, no. 2 (1986): 103–13.

De Capdevielle, B. "An Overview of Project Intelligence." *Per Linguam* 2, no. 2 (1986): 31–38.

Decety, J., and J. Grezes. "The Power of Simulation: Imagining One's Own and Others' Behavior." *Brain Research* 1079 (2006): 4–14.

Decety, J., and P. L. Jackson. "A Social Neuroscience Perspective of Empathy." *Current Directions in Psychological Science* 15 (2006): 54–58.

Derry, S. J. "Remediating Academic Difficulties through Strategy Training: The Acquisition of Useful Knowledge." *Remedial and Special Education* 11, no. 6 (1990): 19–31.

Dhority, L. *The ACT Approach: The Artful Use of Suggestion for Integrative Learning.* Bremen, West Germany: PLS Verlag GmbH, Ander-Weide, 1991.

Diamond, M. *Enriching Heredity: The Impact of the Environment on the Brain.* New York: Free Press, 1988.

Diamond, M., and J. Hopson. "How to Nurture Your Child's Intelligence, Creativity and Healthy Emotions from Birth through Adolescence." In *Magic Trees of the Mind: How to Nurture Your Child's Intelligence, Creativity and Healthy Emotions from Birth through Adolescence.* New York: Penguin, 1999.

Diamond, M., A. Scheibel, G. Murphy, Jr., and T. Harvey. "On the Brain of a Scientist: Albert Einstein." *Experimental Neurology* 88, no. 1 (1985): 198–204.

Diamond, S., and J. Beaumont, eds. *Hemisphere Function in the Human Brain.* New York: Halstead, 1977, 264–78.

Dienstbier, R. "Periodic Adrenaline Arousal Boosts Health Coping." *Brain-Mind Bulletin* 14, no. 9a (1989).

Dispenza, J. *Evolve Your Brain: The Science of Changing Your Brain.* Deerfield Beach, FL: Health Communications, 2007.

Dobson, J. *How to Build Confidence in Your Child.* London: Hodder & Stoughton, 1997.

Doidge, N. *The Brain That Changes Itself: Stories of Personal Triumph from the Frontiers of Brain Science.* New York: Penguin, 2007.

Duncan, J., et al. "A Neural Basis for General Intelligence." *Science* 289 (2000): 457–60.

Edelman, G. M., and V. B. Mountcastle, eds. *The Mindful Brain.* Cambridge, MA: MIT Press, 1978.

Edelman, G. M., and G. Tononi. *A Universe of Consciousness: How Matter Becomes Imagination.* New York: Basic Books, 2000.

Edmonds, M. "How Albert Einstein's Brain Worked." *HowStuffWorks* (accessed December 15, 2016). http://health.howstuffworks.com/einsteins-brain1.htm.

Edwards, B. *Drawing on the Right Side of the Brain.* Los Angeles: J. P. Torcher, 1979.

Einstein, A. *Albert Einstein, the Human Side: New Glimpses from His Archives.* Edited by Helen Dukas and Banesh Hoffmann. Princeton, NJ: Princeton University Press, 1979.

Eisenburger, N. "Understanding the Moderators of Physical and Emotional Pain: A Neural Systems-Based Approach." *Psychological Inquiry* 19 (2008): 189–95.

Entwistle, N. "Motivational Factors in Students' Approaches in Learning." In *Learning Strategies and Learning Styles*, edited by R. R. Schmeck, 21–51. New York: Plenum, 1988.

Entwistle, N. J., and P. Ramsdon. *Understanding Student Learning.* London: Croom Helm, 1983.

Eriksen, C. W., and J. Botella. "Filtering Versus Parallel Processing in RSVP Tasks." *Perception and Psychophysics* 51, no. 4 (1992): 334–43.

Erskine, R. "A Suggestopedic Math Project Using Non Learning Disabled Students." *Journal of the Society for Accelerative Learning and Teaching* 11, no. 4 (1986): 225–47.

Farah, M. J., et al. "Brain Activity Underlying Visual Imagery: Event Related Potentials during Mental Image Generation." *Journal of Cognitive Neuroscience* 1 (1990): 302–16.

Faure, C. *Learning to Be: The World of Education Today and Tomorrow.* Paris: UNESCO, 1972.

Feldman, D. *Beyond Universals in Cognitive Development.* Norwood, NJ: Ablex Publishers, 1980.

Feuerstein, R. *Instrumental Enrichment: An Intervention Program for Cognitive Modifiability.* Baltimore: University Park Press, 1980.

Feuerstein, R., M. Jensen, S. Roniel, and N. Shachor. "Learning Potential Assessment." *Assessment of Exceptional Children.* Philadelphia: Haworth Press, 1986.

Flavell, J. H. "Metacognitive Development." In *Structural/Process Theories of Complete Human Behaviour*, edited by J. M. Scandura and C. J. Brainerd. Amsterdam: Sijthoff & Noordoff, 1978.

Flavell, P. *The Developmental Psychology of Jean Piaget.* New York: Basic Books, 1963.

Fodor, J. *The Modularity of Mind.* Cambridge, MA: MIT/Bradford, 1983.

Fountain, D. *God, Medicine, and Miracles: The Spiritual Factors in Healing*. New York: Random House, 2000.

Frassinelli, L., K. Superior, and J. Meyers. "A Consultation Model for Speech and Language Intervention." *American Speech-Language-Hearing Association* 25, no. 4 (1983): 25–30.

Freeman, W. J. *Societies of Brains: A Study in the Neuroscience of Love and Hate*. Hillsdale, NJ: Lawrence Erlbaum, 1995.

Fuster, J. M. *The Prefrontal Cortex*. 4th ed. London: Academic Press, 2008.

Galaburda, A. "Albert Einstein's Brain." *Lancet* 354 (1999): 182.

Galton, F. *Inquiries into Human Faculty and Its Development*. London: L. M. Dent, 1907.

Gardner, H. *Frames of Mind*. New York: Basic Books, 1985.

———. *The Quest for Mind: Piaget, Levi-Strauss, and the Structuralist Movement*. Chicago: University of Chicago Press, 1981.

Gardner, H., and D. P. Wolfe. "Waves and Streams of Symbolization." In *The Acquisition of Symbolic Skills*, edited by D. Rogers and J. A. Slabada. London: Plenum Press, 1983.

Gazzaniga, M. S. *Handbook of Neuropsychology*. New York: Plenum, 1977.

———, ed. *The New Cognitive Neurosciences*. Cambridge, MA: MIT/Bradford, 2004.

Gelb, M. *Present Yourself*. Los Angeles: Jalmar Press, 1988.

Gerber, A. "Collaboration Between SLP's and Educators: A Continuity Education Process." *Journal of Childhood Communication Disorders* 11, no. 1–2 (1987): 107–25.

"Ghost in Your Genes." *Nova*. Produced and directed by Sarah Holt and Nigel Paterson. BBC, 2006. http://www.pbs.org/wgbh/nova/genes/.

Glaser, R. *Adaptive Education: Individual Diversity and Learning*. New York: Holt, Rinehart and Winston, 1977.

Glasser, M. D. *Control Theory in the Classroom*. New York: Harper & Row, 1986.

Goldberg, E., and L. D. Costa. "Hemisphere Differences in the Acquisition and Use of Descriptive Systems." *Brain and Language* 14 (1981): 144–73.

Golden, F. "Albert Einstein: Person of the Century." *Time* (December 31, 1999). http://content.time.com/time/magazine/article/0,9171,99 3017,00.html.

Gould, S. *The Mismeasure of Man*. New York: W. W. Norton, 1981.

Griffiths, D. E. "Behavioural Science and Educational Administration." *63rd Yearbook of the National Society for the Study of Education*. Chicago: National Society for the Study of Education, 1964.

Gungor, E. *There Is More to the Secret*. Nashville: Thomas Nelson, 2007.

Guyton, A. C., and J. E. Halle. *Textbook of Medical Physiology*. 9th ed. Philadelphia: W. D. Saunders, 2006.

Haber, R. N. "The Power of Visual Perceiving." *Journal of Mental Imagery 5* (1981): 1–40.

Halpern, S., and L. Savary. *Sound Health: The Music and Sounds That Make Us Whole*. San Francisco: Harper & Row, 1985.

Hand, J. D. "The Brain and Accelerative Learning." *Per Linguam* 2, no. 2 (1986): 2–14.

Hand, J. D., and B. L. Stein. "The Brain and Accelerative Learning, Part II: The Brain and Its Functions." *Journal of the Society for Accelerative Learning and Teaching* 11, no. 3 (1986): 149–63.

Harrell, K. D. *Attitude Is Everything: A Tune-up to Enhance Your Life*. Dubuque, IA: Kendall/Hunt Publishing, 1995.

Harrison, C. J. "Metacognition and Motivation." *Reading Improvement* 28, no. 1 (1993): 35–39.

Hart, L. *Human Brain and Human Learning*. New York: Longman, 1983.

Hatton, G. I. "Function-Related Plasticity in the Hypothalamus." *Annual Review of Neuroscience* 20 (1997): 375–97.

Hawkins, D. B. *When Life Makes You Nervous: New and Effective Treatments for Anxiety*. Colorado Springs: Cook Communications, 2001.

Healy, J. "Why Kids Can't Think." *Bottom Line Personal* 13, no. 8 (1992): 1–3.

Hinton, G. E., and J. A. Anderson. *Parallel Models of Associate Memory*. Hillsdale, NJ: Erlbaum, 1981.

Hobson, J. A. *Dreaming: An Introduction to the Science of Sleep*. New York: Oxford University Press, 2002.

Hochberg, L. R., et al. "Neuronal Ensemble Control of Prosthetic Devices by a Human with Tetraplegia." *Nature* 442, no. 7099 (2006): 164–71.

Holden, C. "Child Development: Small Refugees Suffer the Effects of Early Neglect." *Science* 305 (1996): 1076–77.

Holford, P. *The 30-Day Fat Burner Diet*. London: Piatkus, 1999.

———. *The Optimum Nutrition Bible*. London: Piatkus, 1997.

———. *Optimum Nutrition for the Mind*. London: Piatkus, 2003.

Holt, J. *How Children Fail*. New York: Pitman, 1964.

Horstman, J. *The Scientific American Day in the Life of Your Brain*. San Francisco: Jossey-Bass, 2009.

Hubel, D. H. "The Brain." *Scientific American* 24, no. 13 (1979): 45–53.

Hunter, C., and F. Hunter. *Laugh Yourself Healthy*. Lake Mary, FL: Christian Life, 2008.

Hyden, H. "The Differentiation of Brain Cell Protein, Learning and Memory." *Biosystems* 8, no. 4 (1977): 22–30.

Hyman, S. E. "Addiction: A Disease of Learning and Memory." *American Journal of Psychiatry* 162 (2005): 1414–22.

Iaccino, J. *Left Brain–Right Brain Differences: Inquiries, Evidence and New Approaches*. Hillsdale, NJ: Lawrence Erlbaum, 1993.

Iran-Nejad, A. "Active and Dynamic Self-Regulation of Learning Processes." *Review of Educational Research* 60, no. 4 (1990): 573–602.

———. "Associative & Nonassociative Schema Theories of Learning." *Bulletin of the Psychonomic Society* 27 (1989): 1–4.

———. "The Schema: A Long-Term Memory Structure of a Transient Functional Pattern." In *Understanding Reader Is Understanding*, edited by R. J. Teireny, P. Anders, and J. N. Mitchell, 109–28. Hillsdale, NJ: Lawrence Erlbaum, 1987.

Iran-Nejad, A., and B. Chissom. "Active and Dynamic Sources of Self-Regulation." Paper presented at the Annual Meeting of the American Psychological Association. Atlanta, GA, 1988.

Iran-Nejad, A., and A. Ortony. "A Biofunctional Model of Distributed Mental Content, Mental Structures, Awareness and Attention." *The Journal of Mind and Behaviour* 5 (1984): 171–210.

Iran-Nejad, A., A. Ortony, and R. K. Rittenhouse. "The Comprehension of Metaphonical Uses of English by Deaf Children." *American Speech-Language Association* 24 (1989): 551–56.

Jacobs, B., M. Schall, and A. B. Scheibel. "A Quantitative Dendritic Analysis of Wernickes Area in Humans: Gender, Hemispheric and Environmental Factors." *Journal of Comparative Neurology* 327, no. 1 (1993): 97–111.

Jacobs, B. L., et al. "Depression and the Birth and Death of Brain Cells." *American Scientist* 88, no. 4 (2000): 340–46.

Jensen, A. *Bias in Mental Testing*. New York: Free Press, 1980.

Jensen, E. *Brain-Based Learning and Teaching*. South Africa: Process Graphix, 1995.

Johnson, D. W., R. T. Johnson, and E. Holubec. *Circles of Learning: Cooperation in the Classroom*. Edina, MN: Interaction Book Company, 1986.

Johnson, J. M. "A Case History of Professional Evolution from SLP to Communication Instructor." *Journal of Childhood Communication Disorders* 11, no. 4 (1987): 225–34.

Jorgensen, C. C., and W. Kintsch. "The Role of Imagery in the Evaluation of Sentences." *Cognitive Psychology* 4 (1973): 110–16.

Jouvet, M. "Working on a Dream." *Nature Neuroscience* 12 (2009): 811.

Kagan, A., and M. Saling. *An Introduction to Luria's Aphasiology Theory and Application*. Johannesburg, South Africa: Witwatersrand University Press, 1988.

Kalivas, P. W., and N. D. Volkow. "The Neural Basis of Addiction: A Pathology of Motivation and Choice." *American Journal of Psychiatry* 162 (2005): 1403–13.

Kandel, E. R. *In Search of Memory: The Emergence of a New Science of Mind*. New York: W. W. Norton, 2006.

———. "The Molecular Biology of Memory Storage: A Dialog Between Genes and Synapses." Nobel Lecture, December 8, 2000. http://nobelprize.org/nobel_prizes/medicine/laureates/2000/kandel-lecture.pdf.

———. "A New Intellectual Framework for Psychiatry." *American Journal of Psychiatry* 155, no. 4 (1998): 457–69.

Kandel, E. R., J. H. Schwartz, and T. M. Jessell, eds. *Principles of Neural Science*. 4th ed. New York: McGraw-Hill, 2000.

Kane, D. "How Your Brain Handles Love and Pain." *NBCNews.com*, February 19, 2004. http://www.msnbc.msn.com/id/4313263.

Kaniels, S., and R. Feuerstein. "Special Needs of Children with Learning Difficulties." *Oxford Review of Education* 15, no. 2 (1989): 165–79.

Kaplan-Solms, K., and M. Solms. *Clinical Studies in Neuro-Psychoanalysis*. New York: Karnac, 2002.

Kazdin, A. E. "Covert Modelling, Imagery Assessment and Assertive Behaviour." *Journal of Consulting and Clinical Psychology* 43 (1975): 716–24.

Kimura, D. "The Asymmetry of the Human Brain." *Scientific American* 228, no. 3 (1973): 70–80.

———. "Sex Differences in the Brain." *Scientific American* 267, no. 3 (September 1992): 119–25.

King, D. F., and K. S. Goodman. "Whole Language Learning, Cherishing Learners and Their Language." *Language, Speech and Hearing Sciences in Schools* 21 (1990): 221–29.

Kintsch, W. "Learning from Text, Levels of Comprehension, or Why Anyone Would Read a Story Anyway?" *Poetics* 9 (1980): 87–98.

Kline, P. *Everyday Genius*. Arlington, VA: Great Ocean Publishers, 1990.

Kluger, J. "The Biology of Belief," *Time*, February 12, 2009. http://content.time.com/time/magazine/article/0,9171,1879179,00.html.

Knowles, M. *The Adult Learner: A Neglected Species*. Houston: Gulf Publishing Company, 1990.

Kopp, M. S., and J. Rethelyi. "Where Psychology Meets Physiology: Chronic Stress and Premature Mortality—The Central-Eastern European Health Paradox." *Brain Research Bulletin* 62 (2004): 351–67.

Kosslyn, S. M., and O. Koenig. *Wet Mind: The New Cognitive Neuroscience*. New York: Free Press, 1995.

Kruszelnicki, Karl S. "Einstein Failed School." *ABC Science* (June 23, 2004). http://www.abc.net.au/science/articles/2004/06/23/1115185.htm.

Kubzansky, L. D., et al. "Is Worrying Bad for Your Heart? A Prospective Study of Worry and Coronary Heart Disease in the Normative Aging Study." *Circulation* 94 (1997): 818–24.

LaHaye, T., and D. Noebel. *Mind Siege: The Battle for Truth in the New Millennium.* Nashville: Word Publishing, 2000.

Larsson, G., and B. Starrin. "Effect of Relaxation Training on Verbal Ability, Sequential Thinking, and Spatial Ability." *Journal of the Society of Accelerative Learning and Teaching* 13, no. 2 (1988): 147–59.

Lazar, C. "A Review and Appraisal of Current Information on Speech/Language Alternative Service Delivery Models in Schools." *Communiphon* 308 (1994): 8–11.

Lazar, S. W., and C. E. Kerr. "Meditation Experience Is Associated with Increased Cortical Thickness." *NeuroReport* 16, no. 17 (2005): 189–97.

Lea, L. *Wisdom: Don't Live Life without It.* Guilford, Surrey, UK: Highland Books, 1980.

Leaf, C. M. "An Altered Perception of Learning: Geodesic Learning." *Therapy Africa* 1 (October 1997): 7.

———. "An Altered Perception of Learning: Geodesic Learning: Part 2." *Therapy Africa* 2, no. 1 (January/February 1998): 4.

———. "The Development of a Model for Geodesic Learning: The Geodesic Information Processing Model." *The South African Journal of Communication Disorders* 44 (1997): 53–70.

———. "Evaluation and Remediation of High School Children's Problems Using the Mind Mapping Therapeutic Approach." *Remedial Teaching* 7/8 (September 1992).

———. "The Mind Mapping Approach (MMA): Open the Door to Your Brain Power: Learn How to Learn." *Transvaal Association of Educators Journal* (TAT), 1993.

———. "The Mind Mapping Approach: A Model and Framework for Geodesic Learning." Unpublished DPhil dissertation, University of Pretoria, South Africa, 1997.

———. "Mind Mapping as a Therapeutic Intervention Technique." Unpublished workshop manual, 1985.

———. "Mind Mapping as a Therapeutic Technique." *Communiphon* 296 (1989): 11–15. South African Speech-Language-Hearing Association.

————. "Mind Mapping: A Therapeutic Technique for Closed Head Injury." Master's dissertation, University of Pretoria, South Africa, 1990.

————. "The Move from Institution Based Rehabilitation (IBR) to Community Based Rehabilitation (CBR): A Paradigm Shift." *Therapy Africa* 1 (August 1997): 4.

————. *Switch On Your Brain: Understand Your Unique Intelligence Profile and Maximize Your Potential.* Cape Town, South Africa: Tafelberg, 2005.

————. "Teaching Children to Make the Most of Their Minds: Mind Mapping." *Journal for Technical and Vocational Education in South Africa* 121 (1990): 11–13.

————. *Who Switched Off My Brain? Controlling Toxic Thoughts and Emotions.* Revised edition. Dallas: Inprov, 2009.

————. *Who Switched Off My Brain? Controlling Toxic Thoughts and Emotions.* DVD series. Johannesburg, South Africa: Switch on Your Brain, 2007.

Leaf, C. M., M. Copeland, and J. Maccaro. *Your Body His Temple: God's 233 Plan for Achieving Emotional Wholeness.* DVD series. Dallas: Life Outreach International, 2007.

Leaf, C. M., I. C. Uys, and B. Louw. "An Alternative Non-Traditional Approach to Learning: The Metacognitive-Mapping Approach." *The South African Journal of Communication Disorders* 45 (1998): 87–102.

————. "The Development of a Model for Geodesic Learning: The Geodesic Information Processing Model." *The South African Journal of Communication Disorders* 44 (1997): 53–70.

————. "The Mind Mapping Approach (MMA): A Culture and Language-Free Technique." *The South African Journal of Communication Disorders* 40 (1992): 35–43.

LeDoux, J. *Synaptic Self: How Our Brains Become Who We Are.* New York: Viking, 2002.

Leedy, P. D. *Practical Research: Planning and Design.* New York: Macmillan, 1989.

Lehmann, E. L. *Non-Parametric: Statistical Methods Based on Ranks.* Oxford: Holden-Day, 1975.

Lepore, F. E. "Dissecting Genius: Einstein's Brain and the Search for the Neural Basis of Intellect." *Cerebrum.* January 2001. http://www.dana .org/news/cerebrum/detail.aspx?id=3032.

Leuchter, A. F., et al. "Changes in Brain Function of Depressed Subject during Treatment with Placebo." *American Journal of Psychiatry* 159, no. 1 (2002): 122–29.

Levy, J. "Research Synthesis on Right and Left Hemispheres: We Think with Both Sides of the Brain." *Educational Leadership* 40, no. 4 (1983): 66–71.

Lewis, R. "Report Back on the Workshop: Speech/Language/Hearing Therapy in Transition." *Communiphon* 308 (1994): 6–7.

Liebertz, C. "Want Clear Thinking? Relax." *Scientific American,* October 2005. http://www.scientificamerican.com/article.cfm?id=want-clear-t hinking-relax&page=2.

Lipton, B. *The Biology of Belief: Unleashing the Power of Consciousness, Matter and Miracles.* Santa Cruz, CA: Mountain of Love Productions, 2008.

Lipton, B. H., et al. "Microvessel Endothelial Cell Transdifferentiation: Phenotypic Characterization." *Differentiation* 46 (1991): 117–33.

Lozanov, G. *Suggestology and Outlines of Suggestopedy.* New York: Gordon and Breach Science Publishers, 1978.

Lozanov, G., and G. Gateva. *The Foreign Language Educator's Suggestopaedic Manual.* New York: Gordon and Breach Science Publishers, 1989.

L. T. F. A. "Brain-Based Learning." Unpublished lecture series. South Africa: Lead the Field Africa, 1995.

Luria, A. R. *Higher Cortical Functions in Man.* 2nd ed. New York: Basic Books, 1980.

Lutz, K. A., and J. W. Rigney. *The Memory Book.* New York: Skin and Day, 1977.

MacLean, P. "A Mind of Three Minds: Educating the Triune Brain." In *77th Yearbook of the National Society for the Study of Education,* 308–42. Chicago: University of Chicago Press, 1978.

Marvin, C. A. "Consultation Services: Changing Roles for the SLPs." *Journal of Childhood Communication Disorders* 11, no. 1 (1987): 1–15.

Maslow, A. H. *Motivation and Personality*. New York: Harper & Row, 1970.

Mastropieri, M. A., and J. P. Bakken. "Applications of Metacognition." *Remedial and Special Education* 11, no. 6 (1990): 32–35.

Matheny, K. B., and J. McCarthy. *Prescription for Stress*. Oakland, CA: New Harbinger Publications, 2000.

McEwan, B. S. "Stress and Hippocampal Plasticity." *Annual Review of Neuroscience* 22 (1999): 105–22.

McEwan, B. S., and E. N. Lasley. *The End of Stress as We Know It*. Washington, DC: National Academics Press, 2002.

McEwan, B. S., and T. Seeman. "Protective and Damaging Effects of Mediators of Stress: Elaborating and Testing the Concepts of Allostasis and Allostatic Load." *Annals of the New York Academy of Sciences* 896 (1999): 30–47.

McGaugh, J. L., and I. B. Intrioni-Collision. "Involvement of the Amygdaloidal Complex in Neuromodulatory Influences on Memory Storage." *Neuroscience and Behavioral Reviews* 14, no. 4 (1990): 425–31.

Merzenich, M. M. "Cortical Plasticity Contributing to Childhood Development." In *Mechanisms of Cognitive Development: Behavioral and Neural Perspectives*, edited by J. L. McClelland and R. S. Siegler. Mahwah, NJ: Lawrence Erlbaum, 2001.

Meyer, J. *The Battlefield of the Mind*. Nashville: Faith Words, 1995.

———. *Life without Strife: How God Can Heal and Restore Troubled Relationships*. Lake Mary, FL: Charisma House, 2000.

Miller, G. A. "The Magical Number Seven, Plus or Minus Two: Some Limits on Our Capacity for Processing Information." *Psychological Review* 63 (1956): 81–97.

"Mind/Body Connection: How Emotions Affect Your Health." *Family Doctor.org* (May 2016). http://familydoctor.org/online/famdocen/home/healthy/mental/782.html.

Mogilner, A., et al. "Somatosensory Cortical Plasticity in Adult Humans Revealed by Magneto Encephalography." *Proceedings of the National Academy of Sciences* 90, no. 8 (1993): 3593–97.

Montessori, M. *The Absorbent Mind*. Amsterdam: Clio Press, 1989.

Moscowitz, Clara. "Scientists Get First Image of Memory Being Made." *Fox News* (June 29, 2009). http://www.foxnews.com/story/0,2933,52 9187,00.html.

Nader, K., et al. "Fear Memories Require Protein Synthesis in the Amygdala for Reconsolidation after Retrieval." *Nature* 406, no. 6797 (2000): 722–26.

Nelson, A. "Imagery's Physiological Base: The Limbic System. A Review Paper." *Journal of the Society for Accelerative Learning and Teaching* 13, no. 4 (1988): 363–71.

Nelson, R., ed. *Metacognition Core Readings.* Needham Heights, MA: Allyn & Bacon, 1992.

Newberg, A., et al. *Why God Won't Go Away: Brain Science and the Biology of Belief.* New York: Ballantine, 2001.

Novak, J. D., and B. Gowin. *Learning How to Learn.* Cambridge, UK: Cambridge University Press, 1984.

Nummela, R. M., and T. M. Rosengren. "Orchestration of Internal Processing." *Journal for the Society of Accelerated Learning and Teaching* 10, no. 2 (1985): 89–97.

Odendaal, M. S. "Needs Analysis of Higher Primary Educators in Kwa-Zulu." *Per Linguam* special issue, no. 1 (1985): 5–99.

Okebukola, P. A. "Attitudes of Educators Towards Concept Mapping and Vee-Diagramming as Metalearning Tools in Science and Mathematics." *Educational Research* 34, no. 3 (1992): 201–12.

O'Keefe, J., and L. Nadel. *The Hippocampus as a Cognitive Map.* New York: Oxford University Press, 1978.

Olivier, C. *Let's Educate, Train and Learn Outcomes-Based.* Pretoria, South Africa: Benedic, 1999.

Ornstein, R. *The Right Mind.* Orlando: Harcourt, Brace, 1997.

Ornstein, R. E. *The Psychology of Consciousness.* New York: Penguin, 1975.

Palincsar, A. S., and A. L. Brown. "Reciprocal Teaching of Comprehension Fostering and Monitoring Activities." *Cognition and Instruction* 1 (1984): 117–75.

Palmer, L. L., M. Alexander, and N. Ellis. "Elementary School Achievement Results Following In-Service Training of an Entire School Staff in Accelerative Learning and Teaching: An Interim Report." *Journal of the Society for Accelerative Learning and Teaching* 14, no. 1 (1989): 55–79.

Paris, S. G., and P. Winograd. "Promoting Metacognition and Motivation of Exceptional Children." *Remedial and Special Education* 11, no. 6 (1990): 7–15.

Pascuale-Leone, A., and R. Hamilton. "The Metamodal Organization of the Brain." In *Progress in Brain Research* 134, edited by C. Casanova and P. Tito, 427–45. San Diego: Elsevier Science, 2001.

Paterniti, M. *Driving Mr. Albert: A Trip across America with Einstein's Brain*. New York: The Dial Press, 2000.

Perlemutter, D., and C. Coleman. *The Better Brain Book*. New York: Penguin, 2004.

Pert, C. B. *Molecules of Emotion: Why You Feel the Way You Feel*. London: Simon and Schuster, 1997.

Pert, C., et al. "Opiate Agonists and Antagonists Discriminated by Receptor Binding in the Brain." *Science* 182 (1973): 1359–61.

Peters, T. *Playing God? Genetic Determinism and Human Freedom*. 2nd ed. New York: Routledge, 2003.

"The Pleasure Centres Affected by Drugs." *The Brain from Top to Bottom* (accessed December 15, 2016). http://thebrain.mcgill.ca/flash/i/i_03/i_03_cr/i_03_cr_par/i_03_cr_par.html.

Plotsky, P. M., and M. J. Meaney. "Early Postnatal Experience Alters Hypothalamic Corticotrophin-Releasing Factor (CRF) mRNA, Median Eminence CRF Content and Stress-Induced Release in Adult Rats." *Molecular Brain Research* 18 (1993): 195–200.

"Power of Forgiveness—Forgive Others." *Harvard Health Publications*. Boston: Harvard Medical School, 2004, https://www.health.harvard.edu/press_releases/power_of_forgiveness.

Praag, A. F., et al. "Functional Neurogenesis in the Adult Hippocampus." *Nature* 415, no. 6875 (2002): 1030–34.

Pribram, K. H. *Languages of the Brain*. Monterey, CA: Brooks/Cole, 1971.

Pulvermuller, F. *The Neuroscience of Language*. Cambridge, UK: Cambridge University Press, 2002.

Rajechi, D. W. *Attitudes: Themes and Advances.* Sunderland, MA: Sinauer Associates, 1982.

Ramachandran, V. S., and S. Blakeslee. *Phantoms in the Brain.* New York: William Morrow, 1998.

Redding, R. E. "Metacognitive Instruction: Trainers Teaching Thinking Skills." *Performance Improvement Quarterly* 3, no. 1 (1990): 27–41.

Restak, K. *The Brain: The Last Frontier.* New York: Doubleday, 1979.

Restak, R. "Hemisphere Disconnection and Unity in Conscious Awareness." *American Psychologist* 23 (1988): 723–33.

———. *Think Smart: A Neuroscientist's Prescription for Improving Your Brain Performance.* New York: Riverhead, 2009.

"Revised National Curriculum Statement Grades R-9." Policy document. Pretoria, South Africa: Department of Education, 2002.

Rizzolotti, G., and M. F. Destro. "Mirror Neurons." *Scholarpedia* 3, no. 1 (2008): 2055. http://www.scholarpedia.org/article/Mirror_neurons.

Rogers, C. R. *Freedom to Learn.* Columbus: Merrill, 1969.

Roizen, M. F., and C. O. Mehmet. *You: The Owner's Manual.* New York: HarperCollins, 2008.

Rosenfield, I. *The Invention of Memory.* New York: Basic Books, 1988.

Rosenzweig, E. S., C. A. Barnes, and B. L. McNaughton. "Making Room for New Memories." *Nature Neuroscience* 5, no. 1 (2002): 6–8.

Rosenzweig, M. R., and E. L. Bennet. *Neuronal Mechanisms of Learning and Memory.* Cambridge, MA: MIT Press, 1976.

Rozin, P. "The Evolution of Intelligence and Access to the Cognitive Unconscious." *Progress in Psychobiology and Physiological Psychology* 6 (1975): 245–80.

Russell, P. *The Brain Book.* London: Routledge and Kegan Paul, 1986.

Rutherford, R., and K. Neethling. *Am I Clever or Am I Stupid?* Vanderbijlpark, South Africa: Carpe Diem Books, 2001.

Sagan, C. *The Dragons of Eden.* New York: Random House, 1977.

Saloman, G. *Interaction of Media, Cognition and Learning.* San Francisco: Jossey-Bass, 1979.

Samples, R. E. "Learning with the Whole Brain." *Human Behavior* 4 (1975): 16–23.

Sapolsky, R. M. "Why Stress Is Bad for Your Brain." *Science* 273, no. 5276 (1996): 749–50.

Sarno, J. *The Mind-Body Prescription*. New York: Werner Books, 1999.

Sarter, M., M. E. Hasselmo, J. P. Bruno, and B. Givens. "Unraveling the Attentional Functions of Cortical Cholinergic Inputs: Interactions Between Signal-Driven and Cognitive Modulation of Signal Detection." *Brain Research Reviews* 48, no. 1 (2005): 98–111.

Schallert, D. L. "The Significance of Knowledge: A Synthesis of Research Related to Schema Theory." In *Reading Expository Material*, edited by W. Otto and S. White, 13–48. New York: Academic, 1982.

Schneider, W., and R. M. Shiffrin. "Controlled and Automatic Information Processing: I: Detection, Search and Attention." *Psychological Review* 88 (1977): 1–66.

Schon, D. A. *Beyond the Stable State*. San Francisco: Jossey-Bass, 1971.

Schory, M. E. "Whole Language and the Speech Language Pathologists." *Language, Speech and Hearing Services in Schools* 21 (1990): 206–11.

Schuster, D. H. "A Critical Review of American Foreign Language Studies Using Suggestopaedia." Paper delivered at the Aimav Linguistic Conference, University of Nijmegen, Netherlands, 1985.

Schwartz, J. M., and S. Begley. *The Mind and the Brain: Neuroplasticity and the Power of Mental Force*. New York: Regan Books/Harper-Collins, 2002.

Scruggs, E., and J. Brigham. "The Challenges of Metacognitive Instruction." *RASE* 11, no. 6 (1987): 16–18.

Seaward, B. L. *Health and Wellness Journal Workbook*. Sudbury, MA: Jones and Bartlett, 1996.

Segerstrom, S. C., and G. E. Miller. "Psychological Stress and the Human Immune System: A Meta-Analytic Study of 30 Years of Inquiry." *Psychological Bulletin* 130, no. 4 (2004): 601–30.

Shapiro, R. B., V. G. Champagne, and D. De Costa. "The Speech-Language Pathologist: Consultant to the Classroom Educator." *Reading Improvement* 25, no. 1 (1988): 2–9.

Sheth, B. R. "Practice Makes Imperfect: Restorative Effects of Sleep on Motor Learning." *Society for Neuroscience*. Program 14-14 (2006).

Simon, C. S. "Out of the Broom Closet and into the Classroom: The Emerging SLP." *Journal of Childhood Communication Disorders* 11 nos. 1–2 (1987): 81–90.

Sizer, T. R. *Horacel's Compromise: The Dilemma of the American High School*. Boston: Houghton Mifflin, 1984.

Slabbert, J. "Metalearning as the Most Essential Aim in Education for All." Paper presented to faculty of education. University of Pretoria, South Africa, 1989.

Slife, B. D., J. Weiss, and T. Bell. "Separability of Metacognition and Cognition: Problem Solving in Learning Disabled and Regular Students." *Journal of Educational Psychology* 77, no. 4 (1985): 437–45.

Smith, A. *Accelerated Learning in Practice*. Stafford, UK: Network Educational Press, 1999.

Solms, M. "Forebrain Mechanisms of Dreaming Are Activated from a Variety of Sources." *Behavioral and Brain Sciences* 23, no. 6 (2000): 1035–40, 1083–121.

Springer, S. P., and G. Deutsch. *Left Brain, Right Brain*. New York: W. H. Freeman & Company, 1998.

Stengel, R., ed. *TIME Your Brain: A User's Guide*. Des Moines, IA: TIME Books, 2009.

Stephan, K. M., et al. "Functional Anatomy of Mental Representation of Upper Extremity Movements in Healthy Subjects." *Journal of Neurophysiology* 73, no. 1 (1995): 373–86.

Sternberg, R. "The Nature of Mental Abilities." *American Psychologist* 34 (1979): 214–30.

Stickgold, R., et al. "Sleep, Learning, and Dreams: Offline Memory Reprocessing." *Science* 294, no. 554 (2001): 1052–57.

Stickgold, R., and P. Wehrwein. "Health for Life: The Link between Sleep and Memory." *Newsweek*, April 17, 2009. http:/www.newsweek.com /id/194650.

"Stress," *Harvard Health Publications* (accessed December 15, 2016). https:// www.health.harvard.edu/topic/stress.

Sylwester, R. "Research on Memory: Major Discoveries, Major Educational Challenges." *Educational Leadership* 42, no. 7 (1985): 69–75.

Tattershall, S. "Mission Impossible: Learning How a Classroom Works Before It's Too Late!" *Journal of Childhood Communication Disorders* 11, no. 1 (1987): 181–84.

Taub, E., et al. "Use of CI Therapy for Plegic Hands after Chronic Stroke." Presentation at the Society for Neuroscience. Washington, DC, 2005.

Taubes, G. *Good Calories, Bad Calories: Fats, Carbs and the Controversial Science of Diet and Health.* New York: Anchor Books, 2008.

Thembela, A. "Education for Blacks in South Africa: Issues, Problems and Perspectives." *Journal of the Society for Accelerative Learning and Teaching* 15, no. 12 (1990): 45–57.

Thurman, S. K., and A. H. Widerstrom. *Infants and Young Children with Special Needs: A Developmental and Ecological Approach.* 2nd ed. Baltimore: Paul H. Brookes, 1990.

Uys, I. C. "Single Case Experimental Designs: An Essential Service in Communicatively Disabled Care." *The South African Journal of Communication Disorders* 36 (1989): 53–59.

Van derVyver, D. W. "SALT in South Africa: Needs and Parameters." *Journal of the Society for Accelerative Learning and Teaching* 10, no. 3 (1985): 187–200.

Van derVyver, D. W., and B. de Capdeville. "Towards the Mountain: Characteristics and Implications of the South African UPPTRAIL Pilot Project." *Journal of the Society for Accelerative Learning and Teaching* 15, nos. 1–2 (1990): 59–74.

Vaughan, S. C. *The Talking Cure: The Science behind Psychotherapy.* New York: Grosset/Putnam, 1997.

Von Bertalanffy, L. *General Systems Theory.* New York: Braziller, 1968.

Vythilingam, M., and C. Heim. "Childhood Trauma Associated with Smaller Hippocampal Volume in Women with Major Depression." *American Journal of Psychiatry* 159, no. 12 (1968): 2072–80.

Walker, M. P., and R. Stickgold. "Sleep, Memory and Plasticity." *Annual Review of Psychology* 57 (2006): 139–66.

Wark, D. M. "Using Imagery to Teach Study Skills." *Journal of the Society for Accelerative Learning and Teaching* 11, no. 3 (1986): 203–20.

Waterland, R. A., and R. L. Jirtle. "Transposable Elements: Targets for Early Nutritional Effects on Epigenetic Gene Regulation." *Molecular and Cellular Biology* 23, no. 15 (2003): 5293–300.

Watters, E. "DNA Is Not Destiny: The New Science of Epigenetics." *Discover*, November, 2006. http://discovermagazine.com/2006/nov/cover.

Wenger, W. "An Example of Limbic Learning." *Journal of the Society for Accelerative Learning and Teaching* 10, no. 1 (1985): 51–68.

Wertsch, J. V. *Culture, Communication and Cognitions: Vygotskian Perspectives.* Cambridge, UK: Cambridge University Press, 1985.

Wilson, R. S., et al. "Participation in Cognitively Stimulating Activities and Risk of Incident in Alzheimer's Disease." *Journal of the American Medical Association* 287, no. 6 (2002): 742–48.

Witelson, S. "The Brain Connection: The Corpus Callosum Is Larger in Left-Handers." *Science* 229 (1985): 665–68.

Witelson, S. F., D. L. Kigar, and T. Harvey. "The Exceptional Brain of Albert Einstein." *Lancet* 353 (1999): 2149–53.

Wright, N. H. *Finding Freedom from Your Fears.* Grand Rapids: Revell, 2005.

Wurtman, J. *Managing Your Mind-Mood through Food.* New York: HarperCollins, 1986.

Young, Larry J. "Being Human: Love: Neuroscience Tells All." *Nature* 457 (January 2009). http://www.nature.com/nature/journal/v457/n7 226/full/457148a.html.

Zaborszky, L. "The Modular Organization of Brain Systems: Basal Forebrain, the Last Frontier, Changing Views of Cajal's Neuron." *Progressing Brain Research* 136 (2002): 359–72.

Zaidel, E. "Roger Sperry: An Appreciation." *The Dual Brain.* Edited by D. F. Benson and E. Zaidel. New York: The Guilford Press, 1985.

Zakaluk, B. L., and M. Klassen. "Case Study: Enhancing the Performance of a High School Student Labelled Learning Disabled." *Journal of Reading* 36, no. 1 (1992): 4–9.

Zdenek, M. *The Right Brain Experience.* New York: McGraw-Hill, 1983.

Zimmerman, B. J., and D. H. Schunk. *Self-Regulated Learning and Academic Achievement: Theory, Research and Practice.* New York: Springer-Verlag, 1989.

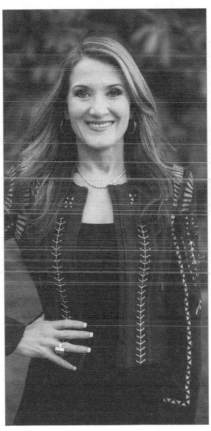
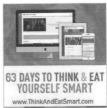
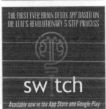
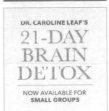
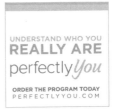

Live a Happier, Healthier Life

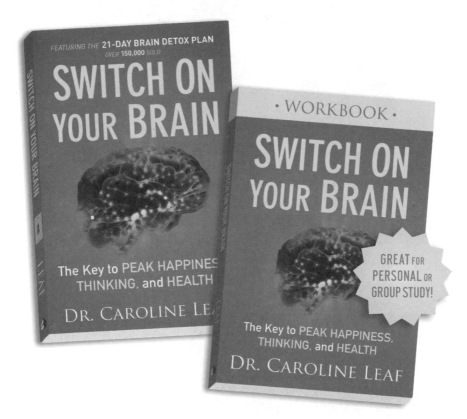

The bestselling book that has taught thousands how to achieve and maintain optimal levels of intelligence, mental health, peace, and happiness!

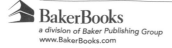

Tired of FAD DIETS, EMOTIONAL EATING, or POOR HEALTH?

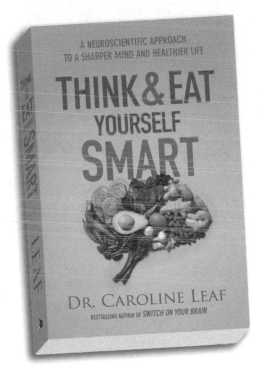

In this revolutionary book, Dr. Caroline Leaf packs an incredible amount of information that will change your eating and thinking habits for the better. Rather than getting caught up in fads, Leaf reveals that every individual has unique nutritional needs and there's no one perfect solution. Rather, she shows how to change the way you think about food and put yourself on the path toward health.

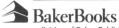

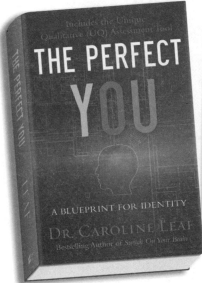
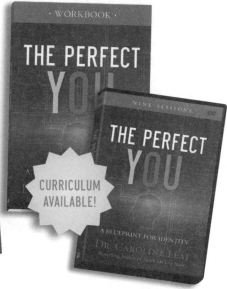